# MANAGED CARE
*made simple*

# MANAGED CARE
## *made simple*
### Second Edition

**Robert A. Baldor, MD**

Associate Professor and Interim Chairman
Department of Family and Community Medicine
University of Massachusetts Medical School
Worcester, Massachusetts

*b*

**Blackwell
Science**

**Editorial Offices:**

350 Main Street, Malden, MA 02148-5018, USA

Osney Mead, Oxford OX2 0EL, England

25 John Street, London WC1N 2BL, England

23 Ainslie Place, Edinburgh EH3 6AJ, Scotland

54 University Street, Carlton, Victoria 3053, Australia

**Other Editorial Offices:**

Blackwell Wissenschafts-Verlag GmbH
Kurfürstendamm 57
10707 Berlin, Germany

Blackwell Science KK
MG Kodenmacho Building
7-10 Kodenmacho Nihombashi
Chuo-ku, Tokyo 104, Japan

**Distributors**

*USA*
Blackwell Science, Inc.
Commerce Place
350 Main Street
Malden, Massachusetts 02148
(Telephone orders: 800-215-1000 or 781-388-8250; fax orders: 781-388-8270)

*Canada*
Login Brothers Book Company
324 Saulteaux Crescent
Winnipeg, Manitoba
Canada R3J 3T2
(Telephone orders: 204-224-4068

*Australia*
Blackwell Science Pty, Ltd.
54 University Street
Carlton, Victoria 3053
(Telephone orders: 03-9347-0300; fax orders: 03-9349-3016)

*Outside North America and Australia*
Blackwell Science, Ltd.
c/o Marston Book Services, Ltd.
P.O. Box 269
Abingdon
Oxon OX14 4YN
England
(Telephone orders: 44-01235-465500; fax orders: 44-01235-465555)

First published 1998

Acquisitions: Joy Denomme

Production: Kevin Sullivan

Manufacturing: Lisa Flanagan

Cover Design, Book Design, and Typesetting by Meral G. Dabcovich, Visual Perspectives

Printed and bound by Braun-Brumfield, Inc.

Printed in the United States of America

98 99 00 01 5 4 3 2 1

The Blackwell Science logo is a trade mark of Blackwell Science Ltd, registered at the United Kingdom Trade Marks Registry

**Notice:** The indications and dosages of all drugs in this book have been recommended in the medical literature and conform to the practices of the general medical community. The medications described do not necessarily have specific approval by the U.S. Food and Drug Administration for use in the diseases and dosages for which they are recommended. The package insert for each drug should be consulted for use and dosage as approved by the FDA. Because standards for usage change, it is advisable to keep abreast of revised recommendations, particularly those concerning new drugs.

Library of Congress Cataloging-in-Publication Data

Baldor, Robert A.
    Managed care made simple/Robert A. Baldor.—2nd ed.
        p.   cm.
Includes bibliographical references and index.
    ISBN 0-632-04378-4
    1. Managed care plans (Medical care)—United
        States.
2. Insurance, Health—United States.   I. Title.
    [DNLM: 1. Managed Care Programs—
    United States.
    W 130 AA1 B17m 1997]
    RA413.5.U5B35   1997
    362.1'04258'0973—dc21
    DNLM/DLC
    for Library of Congress
                                            97-43321
                                            CIP

# CONTENTS

# PREFACE TO THE FIRST EDITION

This book grew out of my experiences in providing health care to my patients in an increasingly managed environment. This work is also a response to the irony of excluding physicians from the initial development of the Clinton health-care reform proposal. Physicians were excluded because it was felt that they had little knowledge of, or concerns about, the economics of health-care delivery. Indeed, there is a fair amount of truth to that statement. Traditionally, little attention has been paid to the teaching of medical economics within medical schools and residency training programs.

In an attempt to rectify this situation, I began to educate myself about the issues of health-care finance, cost-effective care, and managed-care systems and to incorporate teaching of these principles into our medical school curriculum. Unfortunately, there were no appropriate texts or references available for such teaching. Therefore, with the help of two excellent University of Massachusetts medical students, Greg Seiler and Beth Cerce (who have wisely chosen to pursue primary-care residencies—family medicine and primary-care medicine), and the able-bodied research and writing assistance of John O'Malley, we put together a book for our students' use. This book has become an integral part of our family medicine clerkship and we are now moving to incorporate such teaching throughout the medical school curriculum.

While this book will serve as an excellent resource for teaching, it will be of value to any individual with an interest in how we provide and pay for health care. The book reviews the failed Clinton reform proposal and contrasts U.S. health care with that in Canada and England. Various chapters provide an overview of the history of health-care financing, the basic structure of managed-care organizations, and challenges for the future.

As a physician who completed his training in the early 1980s, I never thought much about the financial implications of the care I provided. Now practicing in the 1990s, I am convinced that to truly provide quality medical care, financial factors must be considered. This consideration must involve the same degree of attention as the clinician would give to deciding on the appropriate choice of an antibiotic to treat an infection. This book will provide you with an excellent understanding of the issues involved and allow you to be an educated participant in the still unfolding health-care debate.

# PREFACE TO THE SECOND EDITION

Managed health care continues to increase throughout the United States. Business and industry have fueled this growth with their desire to cut expenses, and it is likewise supported by governmental desires to contain costs. While the managed care principles of providing coordinated, high-quality, cost-effective health care are laudable, a disturbing new trend is the corporatization of health care and the growth of for-profit companies. These companies seek cost savings to support shareholder profits, not more health care. Additionally, as managed care begins to put restrictions on where, when, and how health care is delivered, we are beginning to see a backlash against these initiatives with numerous legislative regulatory efforts.

The need to understand managed care is greater now than ever, for medical students, physicians, nurse practitioners, and other health-care providers. The Second Edition of *Managed Care Made Simple* seeks to convey the latest developments in this rapidly changing field. Every chapter has been updated, and a new section has been added on legislative initiatives. Despite the rapid changes in health-care delivery, one thing remains constant—the provider's privileged relationship with the patient. We must find a way to preserve that sacred trust, while educating ourselves about how best to provide care in managed settings. It is my hope that this book will help to hasten this process.

# ACKNOWLEDGMENTS

I rededicate this book to Kate, my incredibly supportive mate, partner, and best friend; and to my three wonderful children, Anthony, Jocelyn, and Danny, who help to keep me young.

I could not have prepared this manuscript without the expert assistance and patience of Mary Shepard, who works tirelessly to make me look good. A final nod of gratitude goes to my friend and colleague, Michael Ennis, MD, who continually inspires me in my quest for excellence.

## ILLUSTRATION CREDITS

**Cover**       Drawing by Dan Wasserman; © 1989, Los Angeles Times. Reprinted with permission.

**Chapter 1**   Dunagin's People; © Tribune Media Services, Inc. All rights reserved. Reprinted with permission.

**Chapter 2**   Drawing by Dana Fradon; © 1993, The New Yorker Magazine, Inc. Reprinted with permission.

**Chapter 3**   Peter Steiner © 1997 from The Cartoon Bank. All rights reserved. Reprinted with permission.

**Chapter 4**   Drawing by Leo Cullum; © 1994, The New Yorker Magazine, Inc. Reprinted with permission.

**Figure 4.3**  Close to Home © John McPherson/Dist. by Universal Press Syndicate. All rights reserved. Reprinted with permission.

**Figure 4.4**  Drawing by Dave Carpenter. Reprinted with permission.

**Figure 4.6**  Drawing by Frank Cotham; © 1996, The New Yorker Magazine, Inc. Reprinted with permission.

**Chapter 5**   Close to Home © John McPherson/Dist. by Universal Press Syndicate. All rights reserved. Reprinted with permission.

**Chapter 6**   Drawing by William Canty; © 1993. Reprinted with permission.

**Chapter 7**   Drawing by Frank Cotham; Reprinted courtesy of Omni Magazine © 1993.

**Appendixes**  Herman; © Jim Unger/Dist. by Laughing Stock Licensing, Inc. All rights reserved. Reprinted with permission.

**Figure A.1**  Close to Home © John McPherson/Dist. by Universal Press Syndicate. All rights reserved. Reprinted with permission.

# CHAPTER 1

# INTRODUCTION

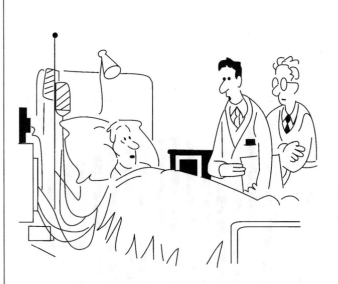

*"We've studied your case carefully, Mr. Twigman,
and you simply can't afford to be this sick."*

Medical care is expensive and getting more so every year. In 1996 alone, the United States spent over $1 trillion ($1,000,000,000,000) dollars, 14.8% of the gross national product, to support the health-care system. Unfortunately, despite the tremendous amount of money being spent, approximately 40 million Americans have no health insurance and an additional 50 million are underinsured. While we can be proud that our expensive high-tech system allows our 80-year-olds to have the longest life expectancy in the world, we lag far behind many other countries in other important health indicators. For example, in 1996, the U.S. infant mortality rate (9 deaths/1000 births) was worse than that of 28 other industrialized countries; the maternal death rate was worse than 18 other countries; and 7% of U.S. babies were born at low birth weight, a rate worse than 30 other countries. U.S. childhood immunization rates are also among the lowest for developed countries, and our average life expectancy continues to rank low (Figure 1.1).

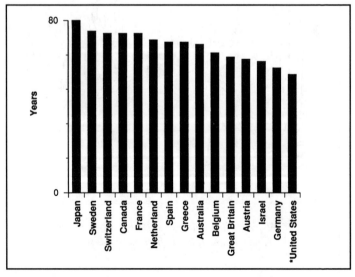

**Figure 1.1** *Life expectancy at birth, both sexes combined, 1990.*

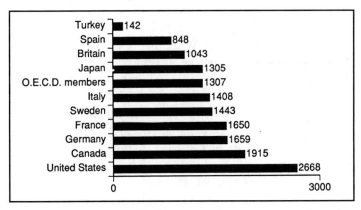

**Figure 1.2** *Comparison of health-care spending: amount spent for each citizen in U.S. dollars, 1993.*

Spending is out of control (Figure 1-2). There are many reasons for the rising cost of medical care. Malpractice premiums and defensive medicine, administrative overhead, expensive technology, unproved therapy, unrealistic patient expectations, and excessive drug costs all contribute to the problem. While there is no single culprit, one fact is clear—physicians play a central role in the system. Despite this central role, many physicians have little understanding of health-care financing and minimal knowledge of the expenses involved in the care they prescribe. It is imperative that, as health-care providers, we educate ourselves about health-care economics and that we become knowledgeable about the care we render and the costs involved.

The United States is one of only two industrialized countries without a national health-care system, the other being South Africa. The reasons for this are complex and involve the interests of a variety of groups. The United States has been debating national health-care reform for almost a century. After the failed 1993 Clinton initiative to reform our health-care delivery system, we were left with a reform based on the private sector "marketplace" in which managed care is the operative delivery system. Managed care has required many changes in how health care is delivered, and, therefore, managed care initiatives have had a major impact on how physicians provide care. While many physicians find this shift to managed care onerous, it is important to understand the underlying philosophy and to appreciate the basic principles and practices of managing care.

This book will provide you with an introduction to medical economics and managed care. You will learn about the history of health-care financing in the United States. In our attempt to push for health-care reform, it is useful to examine both the advantages and disadvantages of programs in other countries, such as those in Canada and Great Britain. The Canadian system provides an especially useful example because of the similarities between the health-care systems of the United States and Canada prior to 1971 when Canada instituted its National Health Services.

Additionally, you will learn about health insurance from the patient's perspective. Chapter 6 explores the costs of pharmaceutical agents, laboratory tests, x-rays, and surgical procedures. Finally, a series of cases are provided for you to work through, and there is a managed care worksheet that you can complete with the help of a preceptor. These cases are meant to be educational, to help you pull some of the book's concepts together, and to provide you with a framework for thinking about how to incorporate cost-effective medicine into your practice. Also, a list of references directs you to further reading and the glossary includes basic definitions that you may find helpful. Finally, the appendixes include answers to the problem-solving cases, some Board Review questions, and tables of common medical diagnostic and therapeutic modalities.

# CHAPTER 2

# HEALTH-CARE FINANCING

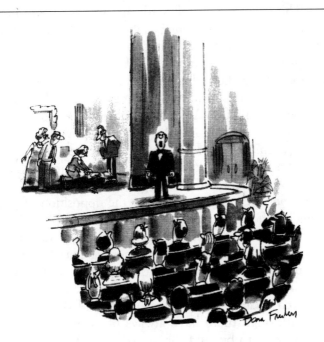

*"Are there several doctors in the house, so we can have a little managed competition?"*

# OVERVIEW

In the early part of this century, patients paid for their medical care "out-of-pocket," much like they would purchase any service. However, with the widespread use of ether and advances in surgical techniques in the 1930s, the medical profession soon had more to offer the public. Progress came at a high price. With the response and demand for these expensive treatments, the first health insurance plan—Blue Cross—was developed by a group of hospitals and surgeons. The early health insurance plans paid only for inpatient care. Physician office visits and medications continued to be paid for by patients who could afford to do so.

The development of Medicare and Medicaid in the 1960s was a critical turning point for the future of medicine. At that time, the United States spent only 5.2% of the gross national product (GNP) on health care. This compared very favorably with other developed countries. Prior to the enactment of these programs, people had little medical insurance. As a result, physicians and hospitals kept fees at lower, more affordable levels. As the government attempted to develop the Medicare system, there was significant resistance from the American Medical Association (AMA) over the perceived "socialization" of medicine. In order to overcome the opposition of physicians and hospitals, the government allowed physicians to set their own fees. Thus, "price setting" by physicians and hospitals was established and soon became universal throughout the U.S. medical insurance system. Essentially, hospitals and physicians charged fees for the costs they incurred in caring for their patients, and Medicare paid the bill, although there have always been deductibles and copayments to be paid for by patients. Physicians were reimbursed on a fee scale based on a customary and prevailing rate formula. This "fee-for-service" system has been under attack ever since.

Health-care expenses increased rapidly throughout the 1960s, and during the 1970s it became apparent that costs

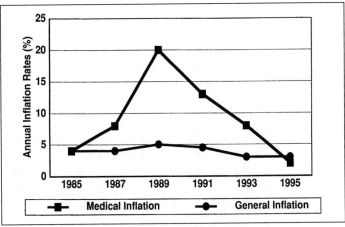

**Figure 2.1** *Annual inflation rates (%), 1985–1995.*

were out of control. Then, annual increases in medical spending far outpaced the general inflationary rates, and in the 1980s and early 1990s these trends continued (Figure 2.1). Today, health insurance is too expensive for the average person to purchase. Fortunately, the majority of insured individuals receive their health insurance as an employment benefit. This "employer-based" financing for health care developed during World War II and has been the standard since that time.

Our employment-based health-care system is one reason for the large numbers of uninsured in the United States. Many employers paying low wages and utilizing part-time help do not offer health insurance as a benefit for their employees. Indeed, the majority of uninsured Americans are working, either part-time or for themselves. Poor people qualify for Medicaid, the governmental health insurance provided for those living below the poverty level.

As costs soared in the 1970s, attempts were made to bring health-care expenses under control. In the mid-1970s, Congress passed legislation encouraging the formation of health maintenance organizations (HMOs). HMOs were designed to operate differently from traditional indemnity insurance plans by moving away from fee-for-service financing. Instead, HMOs were to provide comprehensive care for a flat prepaid fee. The flat fee is an annual insurance premium in exchange for which the HMO would agree to provide all care necessary. This included medications and preventive services such as well-child check, immunizations, and annual Pap smears. Traditional indemnity plans did not cover preventive or routine care, and until the inception of HMOs, patients paid for medications on their own.

It was believed that HMOs would be less expensive, because care would no longer be reimbursed for each service provided. Theoretically, the HMO would seek methods to avoid unnecessary tests and procedures because they would not be reimbursed additionally for extra services. Also, with their health maintenance focus, HMOs would provide less expensive preventive services to their patients, thereby, theoretically at least, preventing serious illnesses that would require expensive hospitalizations and surgeries.

## TRADITIONAL INDEMNITY INSURANCE AND FEE FOR SERVICE

Before the 1800s, medical care in the United States was similar to that in Europe. However, during the last half of the nineteenth century, medicine began to change so that, by World War I, the foundation for present-day medicine in the United States had already been established.

The average physician in the 1800s received training via an informal apprenticeship. The "medical student" was unlikely to see a dissecting room, sit in a lecture hall, or care for hospitalized patients. A small group of physicians held teaching positions in the few medical schools and attended in the nation's few hospitals. These clinicians competed with each other to attract would-be doctors from families who were able to pay high apprenticeship fees. These fees, at the time, were an important part of the physician's annual income.

All care outside of the immediate family (physicians were called only in extenuating circumstances—friends or neighbors acted as domestic practitioners for most sicknesses) was on a fee-for-service basis. Most physicians' chances for economic well-being were small and depended on their ability to attract and hold a sufficient number of fee-paying families.

The physician's bills tended to be kept under the name of the head of the family, and entries included the patient's wife, children, extended family, and servants, if any. Each visit occasioned a separate charge, although bills tended to be settled on an annual basis. Such bills were often ignored until an estate was settled and then were usually paid at a fraction of the cost. Physicians often received payment or partial payment "in-kind." Bushels of wheat, firewood, or days of work at the physician's residence would serve to compensate the physician for his services.

Home visits were the primary method for providing care through the 1800s. A survey published in 1873 revealed only 178 hospitals in the United States. However, by 1923, only 50 years later, there were 6830 hospitals. This, coupled with the development of office practice in the early 1900s, changed the economics of medicine. Office practice was a way of economizing time and resources. The fee for an ordinary office visit was generally less than the customary fee for a house call, but being able to see and treat a half dozen patients during the time it would take to visit one patient increased the physician's income.

The increase in the numbers of hospitals and the development of office practice led to an increasing number of specialists. These physicians had hospital admission privileges in order to achieve more successful treatments for their patients. The older general practitioner was shut out from these privileges and suffered a loss of patient volume and income, especially in urban areas. This, compounded by the problem of too many physicians for those able to pay, caused a number of general practitioners to turn to "lodge practice." This term applied to a form of prepaid health care as opposed to fee-for-service care. The major patient groups that contracted for these physicians were lodges, fraternal organizations, and workers in factories, shops, and mines. The AMA and county medical societies strongly opposed such contract practice.

In an effort to encourage and maintain fee for service, local medical societies began adopting fee tables. These started out as a guide to minimum charges but later became binding on member physicians in a number of medical societies. Fee for service continued as the basic type of physician charges during the twentieth century.

Patients of present-day fee-for-service physicians usually are members of a traditional indemnity insurance plan. Under an indemnity plan the patient incurs medical expenses, pays the bills, and then submits a claim for reimbursement to his or her insurance company. Alternatively, the physician will submit a claim to the insurance company on the patient's behalf and then bill the patient for any balance due after the insurance company has paid its portion of the bill. These traditional indemnity plans are generally the business of private insurance companies, such as John Hancock, Prudential, and Blue Cross/Blue Shield. The plans try to control medical costs by setting fixed limits on reimbursement for specific services or by stipulating that the patient (subscriber) pay an initial deductible and ongoing share of the cost. Thus, indemnity plans attempt to limit costs by constraining the consumer and, to a certain degree the provider, while providing a free choice of physician and hospital.

To *indemnify* is to protect from loss or damage; therefore, traditionally, these plans provided coverage only for inpatient care and emergency service. They did not cover office visits, prescription drugs, preventive health care, routine physicals, or most outpatient services. Recently, indemnity plans have changed to cover some of these services in order to compete with HMOs.

## MEDICARE

Medicare was introduced in 1966 to ensure access to health care for the elderly. Medicare has two parts. Part A covers hospital bills and Part B covers outpatient services, including physician fees. While the private sector has been experimenting with a variety of managed care arrangements in order to keep their employee health insurance benefits under control, the government has tried to control Medicare expenses by changing payment formulas. Diagnosis-related groups (DRGs), assignment, and resource-based relative value system (RBRVS) are programs that have been developed to contain hospital and physician payments. These methods are explained next; however, while they have slowed the increases in Medicare spending, they have not controlled expenses sufficiently. Current plans now focus on further cuts in reimbursement rates to hospitals and physicians, and shifting more of the elderly Medicare patients into managed care organizations.

## Diagnosis-Related Groups

Initially, hospital payments were determined retrospectively by the conventional "cost-based" reimbursement, which essentially reimbursed the hospital for the cost of services they provided. In 1974, the Nixon administration made one of the first attempts at controlling health-care costs by freezing physician fees. However, in 1983, the government made a more aggressive attempt at controlling these costs: DRGs were introduced to reimburse hospitals for the care of Medicare patients. Under this prospective payment system, the hospital is paid a fixed fee depending on the patient's diagnosis. The hospital receives this payment regardless of the actual costs incurred in caring for the patient. While an individual hospital's payment rate is set by taking into account a number of factors, the payment rate for each DRG is determined by averaging the cost of treating a particular diagnosis in the United States.

Indeed, part of the impetus behind the creation of DRGs was the fact that the Medicare administration became aware of great variations in how medical care is delivered in the United States. As a national payer of services, they noticed that the average number of days spent in a hospital and the subsequent costs for similar patients with identical diagnoses varied considerably from hospital to hospital. Thus, a system that pays a standard amount for a given diagnosis, regardless of the charges incurred, was developed. The DRG payment system rewards the cost-effective management of patients. Extra cost incurred by a hospital is the hospital's loss. Likewise, if the hospital is able to reduce the cost of treating a patient, the extra reimbursement is the hospital's to keep.

Table 2.1 demonstrates how one medical center was reimbursed for several patients under the DRG system. As you can see, in several cases, the hospital's costs were several thousands dollars more than the Medicare paid, and in other cases the costs were considerably less than the Medicare reimbursement. The idea is that these costs will balance out in the long run, so that a hospital will break even over time.

Because the payment is based on the patient's diagnosis, not on what resources are utilized to treat the problem, hospitals put pressure on physicians to discharge patients from the hospital as soon as they no longer require the level of care provided by an acute-care hospital (hospital level of care). The hospital may receive the same amount of money from Medicare for treating a patient with, for example, pneumonia, whether the patient's treatment takes 4 days or 7 days.

---

■ **Table 2.1** ▶

*This table provides a partial listing of diagnoses or procedures for actual patients. For each condition, the diagnosis-related group (DRG) category number, the hospital charges for the care rendered, and the actual Medicare reimbursement to the hospital for the specific DRG category are listed. Notice that the reimbursement is not the same as the hospital's charges. For example, the patient with pneumonia was assigned to DRG category 079, which brings a standard payment of $9684, but the cost of the hospitalization for this patient was only $5954. This overpayment is balanced by other patients' costs; for example, the patient who had the total hysterectomy (DRG category 357) accrued $28,592 in hospital charges but Medicare only paid the standard DRG rate of $11,895. The total of these randomly selected cases results in a net loss of over $40 thousand for the hospital. (GI = gastrointestinal; CABG = coronary artery bypass grafting; PTCA = percutaneous transluminal coronary angioplasty; TURP = transurethral resection of the prostate.)*
*\*Costs and payments given in 1996 dollars.*

Since the introduction of DRGs, a variety of changes have taken place in the way that hospitals care for patients. The average length of stay (LOS) in hospitals has decreased dramatically. This, in turn, has resulted in a decreased need for hospital beds, and subsequently many smaller hospitals have closed. These changes have been accompanied by an

## MEDICARE REIMBURSEMENTS FOR HOSPITAL CHARGES

| Diagnosis/Procedure | DRG Code | Hospital Charges ($)* | Medicare Payment ($)* |
|---|---|---|---|
| Pneumonia with lung colllapse | 079 | 5954 | 9684 |
| Asthma with respiratory failure | 096 | 7470 | 5107 |
| Rule out myocardial infarction | 140 | 3435 | 3360 |
| Congestive heart failure | 127 | 5343 | 5358 |
| Upper GI bleed | 296 | 7005 | 5010 |
| Urinary tract infection | 320 | 7778 | 5366 |
| Septicemia | 416 | 6783 | 8177 |
| Chemotherapy, liver | 410 | 2496 | 2734 |
| Cardiac catheterization | 124 | 5219 | 6306 |
| CABG x 2 | 107 | 32,340 | 25,566 |
| Single-vessel PTCA | 112 | 9824 | 10,627 |
| Carotid endarterectomy | 005 | 16,541 | 8137 |
| Hernia repair | 159 | 5464 | 5763 |
| Total hysterectomy | 357 | 28,592 | 11,895 |
| Radical mastectomy | 270 | 4303 | 3581 |
| TURP | 336 | 5635 | 4977 |
| Hip replacement | 209 | 23,783 | 12,644 |
| **Total** | | **$177,965** | **$134,292** |

increased emphasis on outpatient and home care. The DRG system is monitored by a peer-review organization made up of nurses and physicians. They randomly analyze Medicare reports for accurate DRG coding, quality of care, premature discharge, and patient outcome.

## Assignment

While DRGs pay for hospital services, the assignment method was developed in the early 1980s to control the cost of physician reimbursement under Part B of Medicare. As with hospitals, physician reimbursement had been based on a fee-for-service method determined by individual physicians. Assignment was introduced to establish set fees for the various services. Under the federal guidelines, physicians who "participated," agreed to charge patients the fees "assigned" by Medicare. This means that physicians will charge only what Medicare will pay. (The Medicare recipient is still responsible for any deductibles and copayments.) Physicians who did not accept assignment could charge whatever fee they chose. Theoretically, this would introduce competition among physicians and would encourage patients to see "participating" physicians, as their out-of-pocket expenses would be less. Patients would only be responsible for a 20% copayment to a participating physician, whereas, for a nonparticipating physician, they would need to pay the difference between what Medicare pays and what the physician charges.

## Resource-Based Relative Value System

RBRVS, implemented at the beginning of 1992, is the latest federal attempt to control physician reimbursement by Medicare. While DRGs pay for hospital charges, RBRVS seeks to change the way that Medicare pays physicians for their work. Traditionally, procedural skills have been reimbursed at a higher rate than cognitive skills. With RBRVS, physician services are broken down into units of effort, whether cognitive or procedural. The payment formula takes into account the work involved in treating the patient, the practice expenses, the cost of malpractice insurance, and the region of the country.

RBRVS was touted as a boon for primary-care physicians. Early projections predicted that the average family practice physician's reimbursements would increase 16–30%, while, for example, the average ophthalmologist would see a 30% decrease in reimbursements. However, due to cuts in the overall Medicare budget, the average family physician is only reaping modest benefits. The merits of this system are under a great deal of scrutiny, and only time will tell how effectively RBRVS works.

## MEDICAID

Medicaid was established by the federal government in 1965 to provide health care to the poor. Medicaid expenses are borne jointly by the federal government and the states. The federal government will reimburse states between 50 and 83% of what they spend on Medicaid based on a cost-sharing formula that encompasses the individual state's wealth. States set their own rates based on how much they are willing to spend on their percentage of the cost. Each state can determine how much they will pay for services under the Medicaid program, and this is where the most variability exists. For example, in Massachusetts, physicians who deliver a baby are reimbursed approximately $1500; in New Mexico, physicians are reimbursed approximately $900 for a Medicaid delivery. In each case, the federal government eventually reimburses the state for 50–83% of those amounts.

Medicaid expenses have become an annual "budget buster" for many states. In response to this, many states, including Hawaii, Ohio, Oregon, and Vermont, are experimenting with a variety of ways to control these costs. As with Medicare, the main change is contracting with managed care plans to provide health care for Medicaid patients.

## REIMBURSEMENTS (IN DOLLARS) FOR PHYSICIAN SERVICES

| Description of Service | Fee* | BC/ BS* | Medi-care* | Medi-caid* | MHC* |
|---|---|---|---|---|---|
| Outpatient, limited visit | $ 45 | $ 31 | $ 25 | $ 19 | $ 35 |
| Home visit, extended | 103 | 83 | 58 | 53 | 85 |
| Nursing home, extended | 88 | 51 | 57 | 45 | 54 |
| Simple wound repair | 115 | 108 | 69 | 74 | 112 |
| Suture removal, limited | 42 | 32 | 25 | 25 | 38 |
| Flexible sigmoidoscopy | 335 | 101 | 86 | 73 | 144 |
| Colonoscopy to cecum | 1200 | 882 | 473 | 295 | 560 |
| Tonsillectomy/ adenoidectomy | 700 | 362 | 288 | 343 | 408 |
| Tympanostomy with general anesthesia | 380 | 143 | 345 | 189 | 344 |
| Kidney transplantation, surgeon | 5400 | 3008 | 3284 | 2313 | N/A |
| CABG x 2 | 6000 | 4201 | 3783 | 2955 | N/A |
| Hospital care, limited | 42 | 38 | 27 | 26 | 30 |
| Obstetric care, vaginal delivery | 2276 | 1872 | 1084 | 1781 | 1840 |
| Mastectomy, radical | 2000 | 1160 | 848 | 1033 | 1520 |
| Appendectomy | 1000 | 632 | 565 | 404 | 880 |
| Carotid endarterectomy | 3100 | 1783 | 1577 | 1558 | 1200 |
| Cholecystectomy | 1900 | 963 | 891 | 794 | 1080 |

■ Table 2.2
*This table provides a partial listing of representative types of physician services with a fee that is charged by the typical practice. Commercial insurance companies and uninsured patients pay the full fee as charged. Blue Cross/Blue Shield (BC/BS), Medicare, Medicaid, and an HMO-managed health care (MHC) pay less for service rendered, as indicated. In most instances, the fee charged is higher than what the insurance company will pay. (CABG = coronary artery bypass grafting; N/A = not available.)*
*\*Costs and payments given in 1996 dollars.*

## PAYMENTS

Although physicians still charge a fee for services, many insurers pay on a discounted rate. Table 2.2 gives a representative accounting of what physicians in one large multispecialty group practice were reimbursed for care they provided under the Medicare and Medicaid programs. The reimbursements are also provided for Blue Cross and Managed Health Care, an individual practice association (IPA) HMO, for comparison.

# CHAPTER 3

# HEALTH-CARE REFORM INITIATIVES

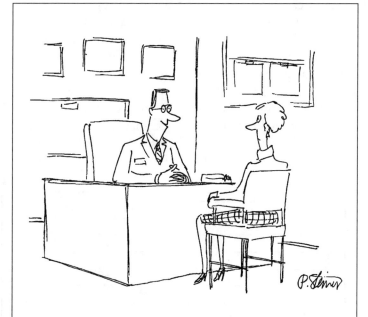

*"Mrs. Bergstrom, because of impending health-care reform,
I can offer you lots of very expensive surgery right now
at dramatically reduced prices."*

## THE ISSUES

The United States has been debating health-care reform for many years now. The three main issues are cost, access, and quality of care. However, the rising costs of medical care have been largely responsible for recent activity in health-care reform (Figure 3.1). While the fee-for-service method of payment has caused some of the problems in the current system, our third-party payment mechanism has also contributed to the loss of control over health-care cost.

Traditionally, physicians and patients would decide on what diagnostic and treatment services were needed and then would turn to a "third party," either a private insurance company or the government, to pay the bill. As health-care costs rapidly escalated throughout the 1970s and 1980s, these third-party payer's began asking why costs were rising so rapidly; they also began to question what they were receiving for their money. Confronted by international competition in all sectors, the comparison of U.S. costs and benefits with those of other countries became a matter of utmost importance. For example, the head of the Chrysler Corporation noted that they were spending more on health-care benefits than they were spending on steel; this cost was three times more than Japanese

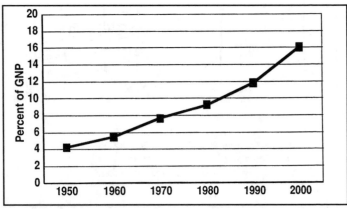

**Figure 3.1** *Health care as percent of gross national product (GNP), 1950–1997.*

automakers were incurring. The government also took notice. Health-care spending through Medicare and Medicaid consume ever-increasing percentages of federal and state budgets. Fewer funds are available for other necessary public spending such as education, nutrition, and infrastructure.

Access to health care became another concern, as many questioned what we receive in exchange for such massive spending. Many Americans go without health care. Approximately 40 million people do not have health insurance and that number increases each year.

Quality is the final policy issue to consider. There is no agreed upon definition of "quality medical care." Therefore, many are questioning the appropriateness and cost-effectiveness of the medical care delivered in the United States. For example, a recent Rand Corporation study in California concluded that 40% of coronary artery bypass graft (CABG) procedures were done for uncertain indications. Additionally, Wennberg has demonstrated wide variations in utilization of health-care resources throughout the United States, with no clear linkage to "quality." Much of what physicians do is untested and unproven to provide benefit. Thus, the debate is beginning to move away from the issue of quality to one of *value*. What do we get for our money? Many studies question whether more health care results in improved health, and, additionally, highlight concerns about overutilization and inappropriate use of expensive resources.

In the early 1990s, the system of health-care delivery was seen as uncoordinated, often untested, and proceeding without any attention to costs. In essence, no one was "managing care." The debate revolves around controlling cost, increasing access, and providing value in health care.

## THE REFORM DEBATE

Over the years, a variety of government attempts have been made to control costs and increase access to health care. Indeed, the Nixon administration called health-care costs a "crisis" and imposed price controls in the early 1970s. In the early 1990s, there was a massive initiative by the Clinton administration at the federal level to reform health-care delivery, and although there was no congressional action, the debate continues.

The debate is raging over some significant issues. One of the major stumbling blocks has been how to achieve *universal access* to care. Many individuals are in favor of a "single-payer" system, which presumably would be much like Canada's system where the government pays all of the medical bills. As the federal government would be the single payer, many people are resistant to this idea. Another way of providing universal access would be to expand the present employer-based system. Currently, this is a voluntary system, with employers providing health insurance as a benefit to their employees. An "employer mandate" would require that all employers provide health insurance for their full-time employees; government subsidies would be provided to the unemployed. The objection to this type of plan is that, in essence, it would be an employer-based tax, one that might be too expensive for small companies and might hurt employment in the long run. While few object to the notion of universal access, how it is to be achieved remains a major political problem.

Another issue with no clear consensus is *cost containment*. Many have embraced the concept of "managed competition," but it is unclear exactly what this term means. Under such a plan, large managed care organizations (MCOs) would succeed and grow, and small organizations would likely suffer. Additionally, to have successful competition in a health-care environment, it appears that concentrations of more than 1 million people are needed. While this may work in large urban areas, most other areas of the United States would not be able to support such a competitive managed health-care environment.

In reforming our health-care system, it is important to separate two aspects of the debate: (1) How do we pay for health care? and (2) How do we deliver health care?

## OPTIONS FOR HEALTH-CARE PAYMENT AND DELIVERY

|  | Public Options | Private Options |
|---|---|---|
| **Payment** | Tax-based system | Individual- or employer-paid insurance premium |
| **Delivery** | Government system like the Veterans Administration | Private/group practice |

■ Table 3.1

(Table 3.1). Health care can be paid for by a public (tax-based) system, such as in Canada and Great Britain, or by a private (individual or employer-paid premium) system, such as in the United States and Germany. Similarly, the delivery of health-care services could be publicly or privately delivered. Great Britain's system is both publicly financed and publicly administered, as the health-care providers—whether physicians, nurses, or hospitals—are government employees and agents. Meanwhile, Canada, though it has a publicly financed single-payer system, maintains a private health-care delivery system. Most providers of care, whether physician practice or hospital, are privately owned and operated. Indeed, many private practices still operate in Canada. However, for all of these only one insurance company pays the bill—the Canadian government.

For more information about the Canadian and British systems, see Examples of National Health-Care Systems at the end of this chapter. Additionally, the programs in Hawaii and Oregon are explained under State Initiatives. These discussions are by no means meant to be comprehensive; rather, they are intended to give you a basic idea of what these systems are about.

# THE CURRENT SITUATION

It is obvious that there are no easy answers for health-care reform, nor is there general agreement about what, if anything, needs to be done. Congress continues to grapple with many of the issues previously mentioned, and it does not appear that there will be any sweeping changes in the immediate future.

The recent passage of the Health Insurance Portability and Accountability Act of 1996 (Kennedy-Kassebaum Bill) may be predictive of future congressional action. This bill makes incremental changes, rather than major revisions, in the system. While the act calls for a new fraud and abuse program for Medicare and Medicaid providers, it also begins to address problems with loss of coverage due to changes in employment. Health insurers in the small group market can no longer exclude employees based on health status. Additionally, coverage must be renewed regardless of changes in health. Those who lose their jobs are now able to buy continuing coverage as individuals; or if re-employed, they may join the new employer's health plan immediately, regardless of pre-existing conditions.

Another key component of the act was enabling legislation for small companies (less than 50 people) and individuals to opt out of traditional insurance coverage by setting up medical savings accounts (MSAs). MSAs are tax-deferred accounts that can be drawn on to finance medical bills, in much the same way that individual retirement accounts (IRAs) can be used for financing one's retirement. However, it is speculated that MSAs will pull otherwise healthy people out of the traditional insurance pool, making health insurance even more expensive for those who need it most. To counteract such concerns, MSAs are targeted for small business employees, many of whom would otherwise have no coverage. Furthermore, only 750,000 policies may be sold annually. Whether this type of coverage will increase remains to be seen.

While the federal government has abandoned attempts at major reform, we will likely continue to see minor legislative

changes at both the national and state lev/
absence of any major public initiatives, the p
"medical marketplace" is making dramatic c_
Managed care has become the dominant theme, driving a
major consolidation of the health-care industry. While
looking for cost efficiencies and profits, MCOs are consoli-
dating to capture larger shares of the health-care market.

Likewise, to compete and develop contracting clout,
health-care providers, particularly hospitals and physician
groups, are merging to become integrated delivery systems
(IDSs). If the current rate of consolidation continues, we
soon will only have 20 to 30 giant health-care insurers, with
100 or so very large IDSs to provide care. The development
of these comprehensive IDSs may obviate the need for insurers, as government and employers could contract directly
with the IDS to provide health care for their beneficiaries.

# EXAMPLES OF NATIONAL HEALTH-CARE SYSTEMS

## Canada

By 1971, Canada had a national health-care program of
universal coverage for all citizens. In 1984, the various programs of the Canadian health-care system were united
under the Canada Health Act. This act established certain
criteria for health care in Canada: reasonable access to
insured services without user charges or extra billing; comprehensive insurance coverage; universal coverage of the
population; portability of benefits; and nonprofit public
administration. Additionally, the training of physicians was
regulated to mandate that 50% of all physicians trained
were to be in primary care.

The national program is based on a series of twelve
interlocking health insurance plans, one for each of the
provinces and territories. Each province or territory is
allowed to determine the administrative arrangements for
the operation of its own plan, providing that the federal

criteria outlined above are followed. The system is financed by the federal and provincial governments.

Each province determines whether to raise its share of the cost through premiums, sales taxes, or other provincial revenues. Physician payment is also flexible. While the fee-for-service system is the predominant method of payment, salaries and contractual agreements are also used. This flexibility allows each province to develop a health plan best suited to its specific needs.

The Canadian system has centralized and streamlined the administrative process. For example, the health-care billing process saves a great deal of time and frustration. There are no complicated insurance forms for physicians or patients to complete. Patients visiting the physician simply turn over their care card, which guarantees them free treatment anywhere in Canada. After seeing a patient, the physician enters a diagnostic code next to the patient's name on the appointment schedule. This code is then entered into a computer, which calculates the charge. The information is then sent to the local Ministry of Health Office. Within 6 weeks, the Ministry sends back a check for the charges.

The effectiveness of the new system has been a lively source of debate over the past 20 years. Certain facts are indisputable. In 1971, health care consumed 7.4% of the gross national product (GNP) in Canada and 7.6% of the GNP in the United States. By 1994, Canadian health-care expenditures had only increased to 8.5% of the GNP, while U.S. expenditures increased markedly to 14% of the GNP. Thus far, the Canadian system has managed to control costs; the U.S. system has not. When pollsters asked Canadians if they would prefer the American health-care system to their own, only 3% said yes. This presents a strong contrast to the 72% of Americans who would prefer the Canadian system.

However, the Canadian system is not perfect. Critics say that the bureaucratic process stifles creativity, and capped fees encourage the most accomplished physicians to practice elsewhere. Patients may wait for longer than one year for elective surgery. The presence of long waiting lists for major operations, especially heart bypass surgery, has been the greatest criticism of the Canadian system. The seriousness of this situation is difficult to determine. In 1991, the Ministry of Health determined that less than 1% of patients waiting for heart surgery died; yet the mortality rate on the operating table is 2 to 3%.

Canadian officials assert that CABG surgery does not save everyone and that some of the patients will die no matter what is done. The Ministry also states that in the United States bypass surgery is often done unnecessarily on patients for whom medications could be just as effective. Other statistics seem to agree. For example, in one study researchers at the Rand Corporation in California analyzed CABG frequency at a local medical center. Of 386 heart bypass operations studied, 154 (40%) were deemed to have been unnecessary. Although armed with such information, the Canadian government nevertheless bowed to public pressure and has taken steps to shorten the waiting lists.

As a result of the Canadian health-care system, every citizen has full health coverage regardless of pre-existing conditions. There are no deductibles, and people choose their own physicians. In addition, Canadian life expectancy is longer and the infant mortality rate is lower than in the United States. Despite the comments of some critics, most Canadian physicians seem to be happy with the system. To date, no mass migration of disenchanted physicians from Canada has occurred.

For the time being, the Canadian health-care system appears to be meeting the needs of its citizens. Its continued success will depend on its ability to respond to more expensive technology and innovative treatments while continuing to provide timely and adequate care.

## Great Britain

The National Health Service (NHS) of Great Britain was established by the NHS Act in 1948. As one of Britain's greatest attempts at socialized legislation, the act provides medical care for all citizens of the United Kingdom.

The NHS has proved to be very cost effective. In 1991, British medical care expenditures were only 6% of the GNP (Figure 3.2).

While many changes have taken place over the past 40 years, many of the basic elements of the NHS have remained the same. The NHS is funded and controlled by the national government. Management of the program is divided into a network of seventeen regions spread out over England, Scotland, Wales, and Northern Ireland. These regions are further subdivided into 221 districts. Each district manages its own hospitals and community nursing programs. Because general practitioners (GPs) are considered independent providers, they are contracted by the NHS. A well-developed primary care system is the most important aspect of health-care delivery in the NHS. More than 70% of physicians are in general practice.

If a patient requires hospital care, the GP will refer the patient to a hospital specialist who arranges the admission and provides care in the hospital. All outpatient care is provided by GPs, and only specialists care for hospitalized patients.

The fixed budget of the NHS often leads to a waiting list for non-emergency care. As in Canada, the greatest problem with waiting lists arises in the area of elective surgical procedures. For the most part, patients on the waiting list have low-risk diagnoses, and few experience acute problems

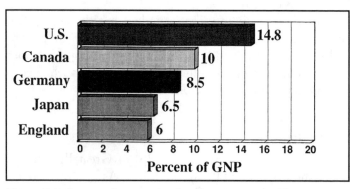

**Figure 3.2** *Percent of gross national product spent on health care, 1991.*

while waiting for their surgery. The greatest criticism made is that a substantial number of patients have reduced functional capacity and quality of life while waiting for care. Those who can afford private supplemental insurance are less likely to wait for elective surgery. With their supplemental insurance, patients can have the operation performed in the private sector. Statistics show that more than 13% of elective operations and 7 to 8% of hospitalizations are paid for by supplemental coverage.

Recently, many questions about the quality of care in the NHS have surfaced. A study done in 1988 in England examined the satisfaction of patients with their medical care. The general level of satisfaction with family physicians was 95%, but specific questions revealed areas of dissatisfaction. For example, 38% of people surveyed felt they could not discuss their personal problems with their physicians, 50% were unhappy with the amount of information they received about health and lifestyle issues; and many felt that their GP did not spend enough time with them. The same pattern was seen in the assessment of patient satisfaction with hospital care. The rate of general satisfaction was 83%, but more detailed questions uncovered patients' concerns. Patients were unhappy with accessibility, hospital organization and facilities, and issues of communication and interpersonal aspects of care.

Additional concerns over inefficiency and ineffectiveness led to reforms legislated by the NHS Act of 1990. These reforms have been directed toward developing policies that encourage improved quality and efficiency.

Interestingly, the NHS is beginning to take on many features of managed care practice, including capitated payments. This is via a program known as "fund-holding." GPs decide how to allocate approximately 20% of the NHS budget in the care of patients. However, if a GP underspends the budgeted amount, the extra money is not kept by the GP. Instead, it is spent on practice improvements or on additional patient services. GPs who overspend their budgets are not at risk (i.e., they are not personally responsible for covering the additional costs).

However, the panel of patients for whom they are responsible may experience longer waiting times for elective procedures and other services.

GPs decide how to spend money on staff, drugs, elective procedures, and nursing home services. The services are purchased from various hospitals, which are organized as NHS Trusts. GPs have the ability to move resources around to those willing and able to deliver services at the best price. Thus, GPs become the patients' advocates by introducing competition into the NHS system.

Expanding on this concept of GP fund-holding is a new pilot program called "total purchasing." This program brings together a large group of GPs to decide how to allocate their combined NHS budgets to care for their assigned patients. For example, one group has a budget of $48 million dollars and responsibility for the total care of 78,000 patients. Thus, the partnership must decide where to get the best value in terms of highest quality and lowest cost for its members, very much like a large group model HMO with a capitated budget in the United States. One significant difference is that the GPs manipulate their budgets only and do not have access to the cash.

Future considerations include possible expansion of the fund-holding concept to specialists, or to the development of GP and specialist teams. Another likely development will be adding risk to those physicians who overspend their budgets.

While the United States looks to other countries for ideas and possible solutions to its health-care delivery problems, many other countries look to the United States for solutions to their problems.

## STATE INITIATIVES

### Hawaii

Since 1974, Hawaii has required employers to pick up the cost of insurance premiums for anyone working more than 20 hours per week. This is known as an *employer-mandate program.* For those not covered by their employer, Medicare, or Medicaid, a state-subsidized program provides care on a sliding-fee basis. This plan allows Hawaii to spend less than 9% of its gross state product on health care. The savings are attributed to the universal coverage that allows patients to receive care in a physician's office, thereby avoiding expensive emergency room care. Moreover, with this universal coverage, people typically do not put off getting care until a problem becomes critical and more expensive to treat. Supporters point to this fact as an example of the benefits of universal access: it serves secondarily as a cost-containment technique.

## Oregon

One of the more controversial state plans that has been developed is in Oregon, which is attempting to radically change health care and the allocation of Medicaid dollars. The Oregon Health Decisions project was established in 1982 to involve the public in resolving problems facing the state's health-care system. More than 300 meetings, involving more than 500 citizens, were held to discuss issues such as personal autonomy, disease prevention, access, cost control, and rationing.

A Health Services Commission worked to establish and revise a Medicaid benefits priority list; this was not an easy task. The commission was made up of physicians, nurses, medical care consumers, and social workers. The list prioritizing care to be provided was developed by incorporating community concerns and cost-benefit data. Table 3.2 outlines the basic rankings for prioritizing care under the Oregon initiative. The most significant benefit of the bill was to expand Medicaid coverage to all individuals living at or below the poverty level, while previously only people living below 58% of the poverty level were covered.

Under the new system, Oregon enrolls everyone eligible for Medicaid but restricts access to treatments below a certain cutoff on the benefits priority list. The cutoff point changes annually, depending on the availability of funds.

## OREGON BASIC HEALTH SERVICE PROGRAM

### "Essential" Services

1. Acute fatal; prevents death, full recovery expected.
   Examples: Repair of deep, open wound of neck. Appendectomy for appendicitis. Medical therapy for myocarditis.
2. Maternity care (including care for newborn in first 28 days of life).
   Examples: Obstetric care for pregnancy. Medical therapy for drug reactions and intoxications specific to newborn. Medical therapy for low-birth-weight babies.
3. Acute fatal; prevents death, without full recovery.
   Examples: Surgical treatment for head injury with prolonged loss of consciousness. Medical therapy for acute bacterial meningitis. Reduction of an open fracture of a joint.
4. Preventive care for children.
   Examples: Immunizations. Medical therapy for streptococcal sore throat and scarlet fever (reduces disability, prevents spread). Screening for specific problems such as vision or hearing problems, or anemia.
5. Chronic potentially fatal; improves life span and quality of well-being (QWB).
   Examples: Medical therapy for type I diabetes mellitus or asthma. Surgical treatment for cancer of the uterus.
6. Reproductive services (excluding maternity and infertility).
   Examples: Contraceptive management, vasectomy, tubal ligation.
7. Comfort care.
   Examples: Palliative therapy for conditions in which death is imminent.
8. Preventive dental (children and adults).
   Example: Cleaning and fluoride.
9. Preventive care for adults.
   Examples: Mammograms; blood pressure screening; medical therapy for primary tuberculosis.

| **"Very Important" Services** |
| --- |

**10.** Acute nonfatal; return to previous health.
Examples: Medical therapy for acute thyroiditis, vaginitis.
Restorative dental service for dental caries.

**11.** Chronic nonfatal; one-time treatment improves QWB.
Examples: Hip replacement. Laser surgery for diabetic
retinopathy. Medical therapy for rheumatic fever.

**12.** Acute nonfatal; without return to previous health.
Examples: Relocation of dislocation of elbow. Arthro-
scopic repair of knee. Repair of corneal laceration.

**13.** Chronic nonfatal; repetitive treatment improves QWB.
Examples: Medical therapy for chronic sinusitis, migraine,
psoriasis.

| **Services "Valuable to Certain Individuals"** |
| --- |

**14.** Acute nonfatal; expedites recovery.
Examples: Medical therapy for diaper rash, acute conjunc-
tivitis, acute pharyngitis.

**15.** Infertility services.
Examples: Medical therapy for anovulation; microsurgery
for tubal disease; in vitro fertilization.

**16.** Preventive care for adults.
Examples: Dipstick urinalysis for hematuria in adults less
than 60 years old. Sigmoidoscopy for persons less than 40
years old. Screening of nonpregnant adults for type I diabetes mellitus.

**17.** Fatal or nonfatal; minimal or no improvement in QWB
(non-self-limited).
Examples: Repair fingertip avulsion. Medical therapy for
gallstones without cholecystitis. Medical therapy for warts.

■ **Table 3.2**
*Source: Bowling A. Management. Setting priorities in health: the Oregon
experiment. Nurs Stand 1992;6:28–30.*

The Oregon plan creates a variety of potential problems for physicians. Physicians have to treat Medicaid patients according to a list of acceptable treatments. Unfortunately, the list excludes treatments of many common problems such as back pain, cold symptoms, skin rashes, and throat problems. Denying care may undermine the physician-patient relationship. In such cases, physicians may be torn between their ethical duties to patients and the limitations imposed on them by the state. This dilemma pressures physicians to diagnose a condition covered by the list instead of an excluded condition.

Early indications from Oregon demonstrate many positive aspects of the plan. An additional 130,000 individuals are now covered by insurance, the majority being families with children. Emergency room usage has fallen by several percentage points. Hospital charity and bad debt has also decreased dramatically. Physicians seem to have integrated the priority list into their practices. However, diagnoses that fall "below the line" can be frustrating to treat, and the line changes annually depending on the state budget.

# CHAPTER 4

# MANAGED CARE

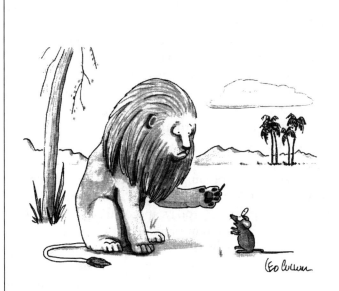

*"I'd like to help you, but you're in a different HMO."*

# ROOTS

**W**hile the need to control health-care costs has fueled the rapid rise in managed care, the basic principles of "pre-paid" health care have been around for some time, dating back to the 1920s. Several factors, including development of the group-practice model and the rise of specialty care played a role in the development of prepaid care.

The transition from general practitioner to medical specialist was made during the twentieth century with relative ease. At the beginning of World War II, only 25% of all physicians were specialists. At the end of the war, nearly two-thirds of the physicians leaving the armed forces entered specialty residency training by using their G.I. Bill's educational benefits, with the result being that by the 1960s some 70% of physicians were specialists.

With this development, there also began a significant shift from private to group practice. *Group practice* is defined by the American Medical Association (AMA) as "three or more physicians who deliver patient care, make joint use of equipment and personnel, and divide income by a prearrangement formula." Managed care is currently fueling the growth of large group practices, as individual practitioners and small groups are less capable of negotiating managed care contracts. Additionally, the increasing supply of physicians, coupled with the selective contracting of managed care organizations (MCOs), is forcing new physicians to become employees to avoid the risks of starting a private practice. Today, approximately one-half of all physicians are in a group practice, with more than 60% of them in multispecialty settings.

At the beginning of the twentieth century, physicians in private practice almost always billed the patient on a fee-for-service basis. That is, they charged a fee for each service or procedure provided. Although prepaid group practice began during the second quarter of the twentieth century, the early growth of managed care delivery was relatively slow.

"Managed care" is a term that has come into common usage during the past few years. Its definition is not universally agreed upon, but it is usually understood to mean a method of providing prepaid health-care services within a defined network of health-care providers, who are given the responsibility to manage and provide quality, cost-effective care.

Managed care was advanced by action of the federal government through the enactment of Medicare and Medicaid laws in 1965 and the passage of the HMO (health maintenance organization) Act of 1973. This health-care legislation expanded the concept of "prepaid practice" and laid the groundwork for increased control of medical care delivery by third-party payers through government-mandated regulations of health-care service. Additionally, the HMO Act enabled managed care plans to increase in number and to expand enrollments through health-care programs financed by grants, contracts, and loans.

Strong support for managed care programs came from both business and government because it was believed that the third party (i.e., MCOs) would control by playing a more responsible role in managing care. In this way, services would be delivered in a coordinated, cost-effective manner; that is, by providing the right care, at the right time, and in the right place. Overall, it was believed, health-care costs would decrease as MCOs participated in free-market competition with traditional fee-for-service providers. Patients are now just beginning to see the positive effects of this competition via lower insurance premiums (Figure 4.1).

## GROWTH AND DEVELOPMENT

Although supported by recent legislation, managed care is an outgrowth of the private sector, dating back close to 70 years.

The year 1929 marked a change in the organization of medical care delivery in the United States, with the establishment of a rural farmers' cooperative health plan in

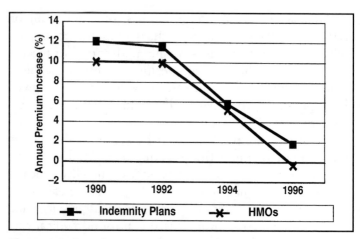

**Figure 4.1** *Annual premium increase (%) for indemnity plans and HMOs.*

Oklahoma. A group of farmers sold $50 shares for a new hospital and provided each shareholder with medical care at a discounted rate. An annual dues schedule was devised that covered the cost of medical care. Also in 1929, two California physicians in Los Angeles entered into a prepaid contract to provide comprehensive health services to 2000 water company employees.

These models led to the widespread growth of managed care plans. Prepaid group-practice plans enjoyed many years of successful growth despite strong opposition from local medical societies. Prominent among the plans founded in the following years were the Group Health Association in Washington (1937), the Kaiser-Permanente Medical Care Program (1942) (the largest, most widely distributed, and best-known national HMO prototype), and the Health Insurance Plan of Greater New York (1947). These plans marked the beginning of managed care, which today serves more than 60% of employed individuals. Indeed, in at least a dozen states, more than one-fourth of the population is enrolled in such plans. Massachusetts leads the way, with almost half of its citizens receiving managed health care.

A variant of the prepaid group-practice plan appeared in 1954 when an individual practice association (IPA) was established in California. A county medical society, fearing competition from Kaiser-Permanente, set up a prepaid foundation for medical care. During the 1980s and 1990s, these IPAs have grown more rapidly than group-practice or staff-model HMOs.

HMOs assumed responsibility for providing a comprehensive range of health services to enrolled populations at a fixed annual premium. Additionally, by combining coverage for outpatient and inpatient care in a single premium, HMOs were able to reduce hospitalization simply by shifting some services to the less expensive ambulatory setting. By contrast, traditional fee-for-service physicians lacked the incentive to reduce access to hospitalization.

A major factor in the success of HMOs is the willingness of physicians to accept financial risk in providing health-care services to groups of subscribers. If HMO physicians incur expenses exceeding budgeted costs, then part or all of the shortfall has to be absorbed by the physicians. Not surprisingly, many physicians resisted sharing in the financial risk of the HMO group practice or staff model. These physicians were more willing to accept the fee-for-service IPA model, even though the fees were often reduced by contracts made between the IPA and HMO organization. The risk was less obvious, and income could still be increased by increasing the number of fees charged.

## ORGANIZATION MODELS

Each MCO has a set of providers (hospitals, physicians, laboratories, etc.). These providers make up the MCOs health-care delivery system. The structure of these health-care delivery systems is vital to the MCO's ability to manage patient care.

In understanding the various models of health-care delivery, it is important to recognize that there are many variations and combinations of the basic models; however, there are generally five basic HMO models: staff, group, network, IPA, and direct contract.

## Staff and Group Models

The staff and group model HMOs have traditionally been called "closed-panel HMOs," as the physicians or physician groups would only provide care for patients enrolled in the HMO. In contrast, "open-panel HMOs," such as the IPA model, allow physicians to care for non-HMO patients along with those enrolled in the HMO.

In the staff model, physicians are employees of the HMO. In the group-practice model, a physician group contracts with the HMO. Presently, both of these traditional models are changing, blurring the lines between open- and closed-panel models.

A few years ago, it was predicted that staff-model HMOs (like Harvard Community Health Plan in Boston) would become dominant players in health care, as they could provide high-quality low-cost care. Although we are seeing increasing numbers of physicians taking salaried positions as employees of health-care organizations, the staff-model HMO is on a decline. The latest rising stars are the network and IPA models, which also provide high-quality, low-cost care but offer patients more choice in their health-care provider. In fact, Harvard Community Health Plan has merged with Pilgrim Health Care and is converting its staff-model HMO into a group-model HMO.

## Network, IPA, and Direct Contract Models

The network model is similar to the group-practice model except that, instead of a single group, there is a network of group practices and, occasionally, independent physicians, contracting with an MCO to provide care for its patients. The IPA model permits the physician to be associated with an HMO without being under direct contract. Instead, these physicians contract with the HMO through the IPA, which is organized around a variety of legal corporations. This is in contrast to the direct-contract model, where individual physicians contract directly with the HMO to provide services.

## Present and Future Trends

In the late 1990s we are seeing a blending of delivery-system models. It is predicted by some experts that most MCOs will evolve into fully integrated delivery systems that contain the features of several models. We hear more now about preferred provider organizations (PPOs), physician hospital organizations (PHOs), and hospital physician organizations (HPOs), in which hospitals and physicians join together to contract with an MCO to provide total health-care delivery for their patients. Another recent development is the physician organization (PO), which brings together large groups of physicians, without the additional liability of partnering with a hospital in these times of declining inpatient use.

All managed care models restrict access to care. They restrict patient choice of physician, specialist, hospital, and medication. Likewise, they restrict a physician's ability to participate in the system. These restrictive methods appear to decrease costs; however, they are not palatable for many (Figure 4.2).

In response to this issue, a new "point-of-service" plan is being developed. The "point-of-service" plan allows patients to receive care outside of the MCO network, but at a cost. Point-of-service plans are more expensive and require larger patient copayments and deductibles than would care within the defined network. Consumer rights groups and the AMA are advocating that these alternatives be required by law for all MCOs.

While the process of managing care is here to stay, the organization of managed delivery continues to evolve. We are bound to see other arrangements over the next several years as the medical marketplace continues to consolidate and reorganize, attempting to find the best model to produce high-quality, cost-effective care.

# FUNCTIONS

In essence, managed care is the coordinated delivery of cost-effective health-care services. The coordination is typ-

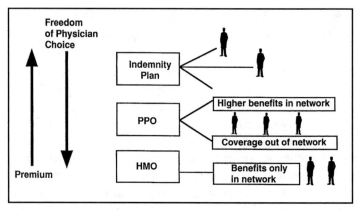

**Figure 4.2** *Managing care controls cost. The arrows at left demonstrate the inverse relationship between freedom of physician choice and amount of premium paid. At right, a comparison of provider choices. (PPO = preferred provider organization; HMO = health maintenance organization. Reproduced from the Group Insurance Commission of the Commonwealth of Massachusetts. Newsletter. Boston, MA, Spring 1995.)*

ically done by requiring every patient to have a primary care physician (PCP) who is responsible for arranging all of the patient's health care. Many techniques are used to help minimize costs. These include: emphasizing preventive health education; restrictive pharmaceutical formularies (see Chapter 6); restricting specialty access to an approved panel of specialists; providing care in the least expensive arena, that is, avoiding use of the hospital in favor of nursing homes, rehabilitation, or home care; and avoiding use of the emergency room in favor of office care. Finally, attempts have been made to encourage cost-conscious practice by providers by shifting from a fee-for-service payment mechanism to capitated payments, which consist of a lump-sum payment for total care to the primary care physician.

## Primary Care Physician

MCOs embrace the concept of the primary care physician playing a central role in each patient's care. Patients are assigned to a PCP who coordinates and arranges for all

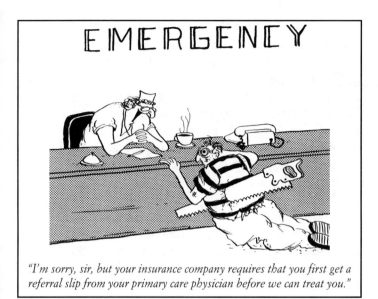

*"I'm sorry, sir, but your insurance company requires that you first get a referral slip from your primary care physician before we can treat you."*

**Figure 4.3**

care (Figure 4.3). This technique is employed in managed health care to eliminate the mismatching, duplication, and confusion that frequently results when patients refer themselves for treatment or specialty care. Therefore, under managed care, a patient is not able simply to see a specialist of his or her choice for care but first must discuss the situation with the PCP who controls referral authorizations for subspecialty, ancillary, and other non-primary care services. Additionally, should the patient need a consultation, the patient must see a specialist who is salaried or otherwise contracted with the MCO in a defined provider network.

## Alternative Care Settings

MCOs also concentrate on controlling how and where patients obtain health-care services. These organizations are particularly aggressive about avoiding use of expensive emergency rooms in favor of the office setting, and about avoiding hospitalization.

MCOs try to limit the use of expensive hospital services via a variety of administrative functions, such as requiring preadmission testing and certification, second opinions, and encouraging the use of outpatient surgery. When hospitalization is necessary, MCOs focus on reducing the number of hospital days by employing utilization review, discharge planning, and case management services. These techniques seek to shift care to less expensive settings such as rehabilitation centers, skilled nursing facilities, or even the patient's home.

MCOs have been very successful in decreasing the hospitalization of their patients. Plans measure their hospital utilization in "days per 1000 patients." The average indemnity plan hospitalization rate is about 350 days per 1000 patients. The average MCO rate is about 250 days per 1000, with some plans as low as 120–150 days per 1000 patients.

## Utilization Management

Utilization management, more commonly known as utilization review (UR), adds a significant layer of bureaucracy to the health-care system. Typical utilization review occurs with an administrative comparison, against a written guideline, of the care being proposed. This process has been a major frustration for many physicians, as payment for proposed surgeries or other treatments may be denied by a patient's insurance company based on an administrative review.

Utilization review can be prospective, concurrent, or retrospective. In the case of a *prospective review*, the insurance company reviews the proposed treatment plan and makes a decision about whether they will pay for the treatment based on their criteria. During a *concurrent review* the admitting physician will often receive notes or telephone calls from utilization review personnel, typically a nurse, questioning whether a patient needs to be continued in the inpatient setting. Pressure to discharge a patient can range from a telephone call asking when the physician is planning to send the patient home, to a more direct statement such

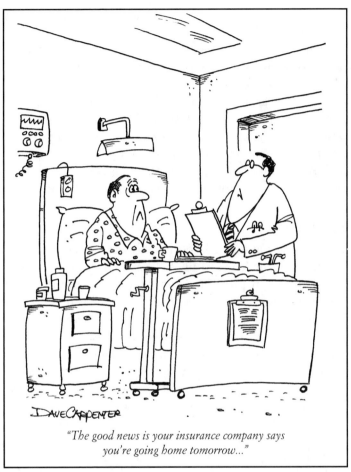

"The good news is your insurance company says
you're going home tomorrow..."

**Figure 4.4**

as "the patient no longer appears to need acute inpatient care, and the insurance plan will not pay for the hospitalization beyond tomorrow" (Figure 4.4).

*Retrospective reviews* tend to be the most frustrating, as an insurance provider, such as Medicare, will randomly audit hospitalizations to make a determination about the appropriateness of the level of care that the patient received. Although a patient may have had an extensive hospitalization with numerous diagnostic and treatment procedures performed, Medicare may determine, after the fact, that these were not medically necessary and therefore refuse to pay the bill.

This can be an extremely frustrating process for physicians, hospitals, and patients. However, it has forced hospital systems to become more efficient and cost-effective by shifting medical care away from the expensive inpatient hospital environment to the less costly ambulatory setting. Unfortunately, one fallout of utilization review and prospective payment under Medicare's diagnosis-related group (DRG) program has been the declining need for hospital beds and the closing of many small community hospitals.

## Guidelines

Some will argue that one positive aspect of managed care has been its challenge to physicians to save scarce healthcare resources by providing efficient and cost-effective care. Evidence-based care concepts are helping in the development of guidelines and "care pathways" that help physicians provide a more consistent standardized approach to the diagnosis and treatment of common conditions. These guidelines are developed based on the approaches medical research has determined result in the best patient outcomes. Unfortunately, for many areas of health care, the medical evidence is incomplete or conflicting, which makes it difficult to draw clear-cut recommendations.

Examining outcomes is a relatively new way to view quality of care. Many providers rely solely upon their training and anecdotal information to guide their care. Indeed, when presented with a similar patient, each physician may approach the diagnosis and treatment differently, yet the outcomes will likely be the same. For example, one recent study detailed sixty-two different diagnostic and treatment approaches for a young woman presenting with symptoms consistent with cystitis. Given the differences in cost for the various approaches, many payers are questioning whether they should pay for the expensive approach when a less expensive approach can provide the same outcome. Many guidelines are developed based on this underlying concept.

## WORKFORCE ISSUES

**W**hile managed care plans seek large numbers of primary care physicians within their organizations, they limit the number of specialists. This has raised questions about the appropriate balance between generalists (primary care) and specialist physicians needed to provide optimal care for patients. Although there is considerable debate concerning this issue, many health-care analysts are arguing for a 50/50 ratio of generalists to specialists, which is approximately the division that exists in Canada. Elsewhere, such as in Great Britain, percentages are much different, roughly opposite from what we have in the United States today (i.e., 70% specialists to 30% generalists). Recent studies have examined this issue, and it has been projected that we have available an oversupply of specialists and a slight undersupply of generalists available to meet U.S. physician workforce needs (Figure 4.5).

In response to such information, medical schools are attempting to change their curriculums to be more supportive of the general/primary care physician. Additionally, family practice residencies have increased throughout the United States in order to provide adequate postgraduate training for students interested in pursuing primary care careers.

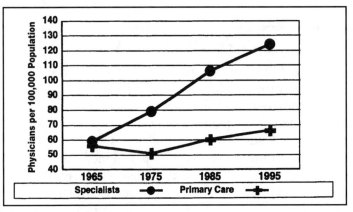

**Figure 4.5** *Physicians per 100,000 population.*

Given the dramatic changes in health-care delivery and the changing needs of the marketplace, some authors have raised the specter of physician unemployment, particularly for specialists. Indeed, in some areas of the United States, particularly where there has been a high penetration of managed care, specialists are having difficulty finding employment and the phenomenon of retraining has become a reality. Some of the better-known programs in retraining have sprung up in Boston, Philadelphia, and San Diego. Given this incredible change in the marketplace, it behooves students interested in specialty practice to fully explore the ramifications of their decision, especially with regard to future employment.

Our health-care system is undergoing a massive consolidation as we move toward integrated systems. These systems seek out large numbers of primary care physicians in order to support their specialty-/hospital-based organizations. While this is appropriate given the current reimbursement structures, the organizations that survive will be those that embrace primary care and prevention and consider hospitalization the system's failure to provide appropriate, high-quality care. In the mature integrated health-care delivery systems of the future, hospitals and subspecialists will work to support the care being provided by the primary care physician, unlike the current structure in which primary care physicians are supporting specialty/hospital systems.

## PAYMENT METHODS

**M**anaged care payment to hospitals and physicians comes in many forms, including discounted charges, DRG or resource-based relative value system (RBRVS) payments, and capitation. Capitated managed care plans are a somewhat radical attempt at controlling costs. With capitated payment, an insurance company pays a medical provider a flat fee each month for every patient who has signed up with that provider for care. Capitated payments can be offered to primary care physicians, specialists, or hospitals and are an amount "per member per month." Interestingly, the provider receives this payment whether the patient is treated or not. While there are many types of capitated payments, a typical primary care physician's payments will also include funds for specialty referrals and laboratory testing. For example, if the physician refers the patient for specialty care, lab work, or radiologic procedures, the cost of this care is deducted from his/her monthly payment. Clearly, this provides a sufficient incentive to avoid excessive use of these services. Captitated payment is only one of the more drastic approaches used by managed care plans, although it is not a new concept; the Kaiser plan capitated payments when it started earlier in this century.

Capitation changes the focus from how much a provider will be paid, as is the case with fee for service, to how much it costs to provide the care required. When a provider becomes financially "at risk" for the expenses incurred in caring for their patients, services become costs, not revenues. Under capitation, if patients use excessive medical services because of inappropriate utilization or illness, those services (costs) are paid from the capitated payment pool, leaving less for the provider. However, by maintaining health and preventing disease exacerbations, less health-care costs are incurred. The physician shares the financial savings with the MCO.

Inasmuch as a successful capitation program is partially based on the law of averages, under this plan it is necessary for an individual physician to have at least 300 patients to control the level of risk and to experience long-term economic success. Additionally, secondary insurance may be purchased by the physician to cover catastrophic episodes. Finally, to further spread the financial risk, physicians are forming into larger and larger groups in order to obtain capitated contracts for large pools of patients.

## ETHICAL CONSIDERATIONS

The changes in health-care delivery have stimulated many ethical concerns. Although there are no easy answers or particular "rights or wrongs" for many of the issues, it is incumbent upon us, as health-care professionals, to be aware of potential conflicts. The most notable areas of concern include capitated payment schemes, the "for-profit" corporatization of health care, and rationing of care.

Under capitation, the physician is rewarded for not providing services; that is, the less a patient utilizes the system, the more the physician benefits financially. Although people consider this approach with great cynicism, it is best evaluated when juxtaposed to the fee-for-service system. Under traditional fee-for-service care, physicians are rewarded for providing services; that is, the more a patient utilizes the system, the more the physician benefits financially (Figure 4.6). Thus, some argue that under a fee-for-service plan physicians are paid for doing things to people, not for keeping them healthy, while under capitation physicians are encouraged to keep their patients healthy and avoid the need to "do things to them."

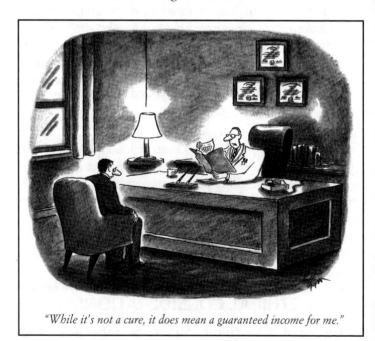

*"While it's not a cure, it does mean a guaranteed income for me."*

50

**Figure 4.6**

Perhaps an even greater concern is the corporatization of medical care. Medical care is evolving from a cottage industry into a large corporate structure. Many of these "corporate" organizations are for-profit, and any savings squeezed out of the system goes to improve the financial interest of stockholders. While profits have always been made in the medical industry, typically, significant amounts of these revenues have been poured back into the system, in order to provide or improve care. Such initiatives include charitable contributions of "free care" or improvement of care via funding of research and teaching programs. Although few would argue against the concept of cost-effective care, there is considerable concern about use of these techniques to generate profit for shareholders at the potential expense of patients.

The issue of rationing has been raised within the context of the changes made to Oregon's Medicaid program, where services are provided based on a severity model, coupled with likelihood of benefit and availability of resources (see Chapter 3 for an overview of Oregon's program). Additionally, rationing becomes a concern when large MCOs restrict patient access to certain types of care, such as bone marrow transplants for breast cancer patients. Rationing weighs individual benefits versus society or public health benefits. For example, in this era of limited resources, should we spend $100,000 to treat a patient dying from breast cancer (with modest likelihood of cure), or on probably futile ICU care for an elderly patient with cor pulmonale from chronic obstructive pulmonary disease (COPD) caused by a lifetime of smoking? Or should the money be used to immunize 5000 children against infectious diseases?

The AMA's Council on Ethical and Judicial Affairs has released a set of guidelines for physicians and organizations—a strong first step in incorporating ethical considerations into MCOs policies and procedures regarding the provision of care. In order to avoid ethical dilemmas, it is incumbent on the physician to attend to each individual patient's needs as appropriate, regardless of the health-care delivery system in which the physician practices. By providing care in a patient-centered, cost-effective manner, we can feel comfortable and confident that we have our patients' best interests at heart.

## LEGISLATIVE INITIATIVES

**R**estrictions of health-care delivery have sparked an angry backlash against managed care. This backlash has translated into a variety of legislative initiatives, primarily at the state level. More than 400 anti-managed care bills were proposed in state legislatures during 1996 alone. Many of these initiatives have dealt with access to the hospital and subspecialty care.

*"Any willing provider" laws* have been developed to counter the restrictive and exclusive contracting practices of MCOs. These legislative initiatives would require MCOs to contract with any provider who is willing to accept the payments being offered. Many specialists are being excluded from managed care networks, and this type of legislation would facilitate their participation in these systems.

*Drive-through delivery laws* have also received considerable attention. Many MCOs refuse to pay for postpartum stays beyond 24 hours for normal routine deliveries (although the better MCOs provide postpartum home care). This practice has prompted a collective outcry from a number of constituents. As a result, many states have legislated a mandated 48-hour stay for these patients. Whether staying in the hospital is more beneficial to the mother and infant than being discharged home has not been adequately studied. Recently, similar legislation has been introduced concerning care of women who have received mastectomies; it insists that they be allowed to stay in the hospital for a prolonged period to recover from the trauma of potentially disfiguring surgery.

*Gag rules* have come under scrutiny. Such legislation prohibits MCOs from penalizing physicians who advocate care that is not covered by the health-care plan for their patients.

Finally, many have argued that MCOs are overly aggressive in restricting use of emergency room care, refusing to pay for emergency room visits if they are deemed not to be true emergencies. The definition of a "true emergency" is somewhat subjective, so legislation has been filed defining a "prudent lay person's" definition as the standard.

While oversight of the new managed health-care industry is necessary, such specific legislation can only continue to frustrate providers of care. Additionally, MCOs are fighting these legislative initiatives, arguing that such laws diminish their ability to control costs and ensure quality. One likely outcome of all these initiatives is to accelerate the movement to capitated payments. Under such schemes, the MCO removes itself from the specifics of managing care, instead putting the total burden, including the cost of care, on the providers.

# CHAPTER 5

# HEALTH INSURANCE—
# THE PATIENT'S PERSPECTIVE

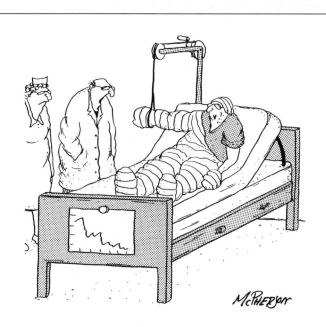

*"Your insurance company is refusing to pay your medical bills due to a pre-existing condition. It says you were already an idiot before you decided to Rollerblade down the interstate."*

Presently, a complex mixture of public and private health insurance programs cover the majority of American health-care needs. This includes Medicaid for the impoverished, Medicare for the elderly, and a variety of private plans for those who can afford them. However, despite this, approximately 40 million Americans do not have health insurance, as they do not meet the requirements for government-sponsored public care, do not receive health-care benefits from their employers, and cannot afford to pay for private insurance. This chapter provides an overview of insurance programs from the patient's perspective, outlining eligibility criteria and cost.

## PRIVATE INSURANCE

Most insured individuals obtain insurance as part of a benefits package from their employer. Employer-based financing for health care developed during World War II, and this practice has increased steadily since that time. Although the employer helps pay for the insurance, workers pay a percentage of the insurance premium. Nevertheless, this is a tremendous benefit, as the overall premiums for an employer, because the risk is spread out over a larger group, are lower than they would be if workers bought health insurance as individuals. For example, for a healthy, young family of four to buy insurance on their own without the benefit of employer assistance, they would have to spend about $5 thousand per year.

While an excellent benefit for employees, the practice of providing health insurance can get very expensive for employers, as they spend thousands of dollars per employee every year. For example, in 1995, employers paid an average of about $3800 per employee for health insurance.

Individuals can choose from a variety of health insurance plans but are usually restricted to what is offered through their employer. Thus, employees may have little choice in the type of health insurance to which they can subscribe; in fact, many companies offer only one insurance plan for their workers.

Insurance plans range from traditional indemnity plans to health maintenance organizations (HMOs). Traditional indemnity plans like John Hancock or Blue Cross/Blue Shield insurance allow the patient considerable freedom in choosing their physicians, whether primary care or subspecialty oriented. However, this comes at a much higher cost than HMO care. Table 5.1 shows the cost of health insurance for one large business and its employees.

Insurance plans limit their coverage and their financial exposure via a benefits package. This package lists the specific benefits and services they are obligated to provide (or pay for) under the terms of their contract with the subscriber. All additional benefits, especially with newly developing procedures and surgery, are provided only at the discretion of the plan's management. The limitation of benefits by managed care health plans has caused concern and lawsuits in some cases. The most well-publicized example has been for coverage of bone marrow transplantation to treat breast cancer. Health plans often refuse to cover this and other expensive therapies as they are still considered "experimental." Most plans exclude coverage of experimental therapies from their benefits package.

## MEDICARE

Medicare is a federal health insurance program for people 65 years or older. Basically, people qualify for Medicare coverage on their 65th birthday, if they meet the stipulated work requirement (i.e., ten full-time equivalent work quarters). The majority of elderly Americans qualify. Additionally, some people can claim benefits on the account of someone who has met the work requirements (e.g., a spouse). Medicare is also available to some people under age 65, if they have permanent kidney failure or if they have been receiving Social Security disability payments for 2 years.

## ANNUAL HEALTH INSURANCE PREMIUMS ($)
## FOR A LARGE COMPANY'S EMPLOYEES (7/1/97)

| Insurance Company | Employee Premium | Employer Contribution | Total Cost |
|---|---|---|---|
| **Indemnity Plan with CIC** | | | |
| Individual | 772.56 | 3360.24 | 4132.80 |
| Family | 1749.72 | 7599.24 | 9348.96 |
| **Indemnity Plan without CIC** | | | |
| Individual | 578.28 | 3360.24 | 3938.52 |
| Family | 1298.52 | 7599.24 | 8897.76 |
| **PPO Plan** | | | |
| Individual | 403.32 | 2285.40 | 2688.72 |
| Family | 936.96 | 5309.28 | 6246.24 |
| **Kaiser-Permanente HMO** | | | |
| Individual | 306.84 | 1690.80 | 1997.64 |
| Family | 743.64 | 4213.68 | 4957.32 |
| **Harvard Pilgrim Health Care** | | | |
| Individual | 356.64 | 2020.92 | 2377.56 |
| Family | 851.64 | 4825.92 | 5677.56 |
| **Healthsource** | | | |
| Individual | 309.24 | 1752.24 | 2061.48 |
| Family | 785.04 | 4448.28 | 5233.32 |
| **Neighborhood Health Plan** | | | |
| Individual | 780.00 | 1812.12 | 2592.12 |
| Family | 816.72 | 4628.28 | 5445.00 |
| **Tufts Health Plan** | | | |
| Individual | 345.72 | 1959.12 | 2304.84 |
| Family | 816.96 | 4629.12 | 5446.08 |

■ Table 5.1

*CIC = catastrophic illness coverage.*

Medicare comes in two parts. Part A covers inpatient care, and all Americans who have met the work requirements are automatically entitled to this coverage at age 65. Part A covers hospital bills and bills for skilled nursing homes. Additionally, Part A covers some hospice care and minimal home health care.

Part B is optional coverage. In order to qualify for Part B, elder recipients must pay a premium for this coverage. In 1997, the premium was $525.60 per year. Part B covers physician bills and outpatient services such as surgery and diagnostic testing. Additionally, it covers some medical supplies and other miscellaneous costs. Most people consider Part B to be reasonably priced, as the federal government pays 75% of the program cost and individuals have to pay only a small monthly premium (about $44 per month), which is usually subtracted from their Social Security retirement check. In addition to the premiums, patients are responsible for deductibles and copayments.

A *deductible* is a predetermined amount that the patient must pay before Medicare begins to pay for any covered services. In 1997, the Part A deductible was $760 per benefit period. A *benefit period* begins on the first day of an inpatient hospital care and ends when the patient has been out of the hospital 60 consecutive days; therefore, it is conceivable that a patient may have to pay more than one Part A deductible during any given year. The Part B deductible in 1997 was $100 per calendar year. Patients must pay this first $100 for outpatient and physician treatments covered under Part B before Medicare insurance will begin payment.

A *copayment* is a certain percent of the physician's charges that the patient must pay, in addition to what Medicare pays. Medicare, although it sets approved charge levels, typically pays only 80% of these charges. Therefore, patients who have Medicare as their insurance are required to pay the additional 20% of the approved charges. Individuals can purchase Medicare supplemental insurance to cover this 20% copayment.

Impoverished elderly patients can also qualify for Medicaid (see next section). If they meet the eligibility

## OUTLINE OF MEDICARE SUPPLEMENTAL COVERAGE

| A | B | C | D | E | F | G | H | I | J |
|---|---|---|---|---|---|---|---|---|---|
| Basic benefits | Basic benefits | Basic benefits | Basic benefits | Basic benefits | Basic benefits | Basic benefits | Basic benefits | Basic benefits | Basic benefits |
| | | Skilled nursing co-insurance | Skilled nursing co-insurance | Skilled nursing co-insurance | Skilled nursing co-insurance | Skilled nursing co-insurance | Skilled nursing co-insurance | Skilled nursing co-insurance | Skilled nursing co-insurance |
| | Part A deductible | Part A deductible | Part A deductible | Part A deductible | Part A deductible | Part A deductible | Part A deductible | Part A deductible | Part A deductible |
| | | Part B deductible | | | Part B deductible | | | | Part B deductible |
| | | | | | Part B excess (100%) | Part B excess (100%) | | Part B excess (100%) | Part B excess (100%) |
| | | Foreign travel emergency | Foreign travel emergency | Foreign travel emergency | Foreign travel emergency | Foreign travel emergency | Foreign travel emergency | Foreign travel emergency | Foreign travel emergency |
| | | | At-home recovery | | | At-home recovery | | At-home recovery | At-home recovery |
| | | | | | | | Basic drugs ($1250) | Basic drugs ($1250) | Extended drugs ($3000 limit) |
| | | | | Preventive care | | | | | Preventive care |

requirements, Medicaid will pay their Medicare deductibles and copayments.

As wonderful as the Medicare system sounds, there are several gaps in the coverage, and numerous private insurance companies sell supplemental coverage programs.

There used to be an amazing array of Medicare supplemental coverage plans available, but this has changed recently, as Congress legislated ten standard plans that private insurance companies can sell to people who want to supplement their basic Medicare benefits. Standard plans are labeled A through J and include benefit packages that range from a bare-bones policy to a comprehensive policy. Under federal and state law, only these ten plans may be sold so that consumers can compare the different policies. Plans B through J add extras, such as coverage for deductibles, prescription drugs, and so on. Table 5.2 outlines the Medicare supplemental insurance options.

## MEDICAID

Medicaid was established by the federal government in 1965 to provide health care to impoverished individuals and, in particular, to families with dependent children, the aged, the blind, and persons who are permanently and totally disabled.

This program, known as Title XIX, has cost-sharing with the states and is administered by each state, operating

---

**■ TABLE 5.2**

*Medicare supplement insurance can be sold in only ten standard plans. This chart shows the benefits included in each plan. Every company must make available "plan A." Some plans may not be available in your state.*

*Basic benefits (included in all plans):*
> *Hospitalization: Part A coinsurance plus coverage for 365 additional days after Medicare benefits end.*
> *Medical Expenses: Part B coinsurance (20% of Medicare-approved expenses).*
> *Blood: First 3 pints of blood each year.*

within broad federal guidelines. The federal share of the program's costs is 50 to 83% according to a state's per capita income, and averages 55% nationwide. To qualify for this program, individuals must be eligible for Aid to Families with Dependent Children (AFDC), Old-Age Assistance, or Aid to the Blind, or Permanently and Totally Disabled, or be elderly (over 65 years) and on welfare. All needy children (under age 21) are also eligible.

Medicaid is a blanket label for fifty different state programs, designed specifically to serve the poor. Eligibility for Medicaid varies widely, as it is determined by each state. However, all states must cover those receiving cash assistance, poor children up to the age of five, pregnant women who are poor and who will qualify for cash assistance programs when their children are born, and pregnant women in two parent families with an unemployed principal wage earner. States also have the option of expanding coverage to special groups such as individuals who become poor due to expenditures on health care.

State flexibility in determining eligibility standards has created wide variation in Medicaid coverage. Some states set income standards below the federal poverty level (Table 5.3); others expand coverage to a categorically needy group. Thus, eligibility for Medicaid is a complex process. Social workers are available in most states to help potentially qualified patients determine for which benefits they are eligible.

## LONG-TERM CARE

*Long-term care* refers to care provided to individuals who can no longer care for themselves. Usually this term is used when talking about nursing home care. The levels of long-term care are varied. Many assume that Medicare will pay for long-term nursing home care. In reality, Medicare provides very limited coverage for skilled nursing care. Medicare Part A pays all expenses for the first 20 days in a skilled nursing facility (SNF). However, for the next 80 days, the patient is responsible for a copayment of $87 per day.

## FEDERAL POVERTY LEVEL (1997)

| Family Size | Annual Income Standards |
|---|---|
| 1 | $  7740 |
| 2 | 10,360 |
| 3 | 12,980 |
| 4 | 15,600 |
| 5 | 18,220 |
| 6 | 20,840 |
| 7 | 23,460 |
| 8 | 26,080 |
| Each additional person | +2620 |

■ Table 5.3

No coverage is provided for stays longer than 100 days. After 100 days of skilled nursing care, the majority of patients no longer need skilled care and transfer to custodial care. A nursing home that provides custodial care is not covered by Medicare, nor is it covered by supplemental policies.

Once Medicare benefits are exhausted, the patient is forced to rely on personal resources to finance care. To receive governmental assistance, the patient must "spend down" assets in order to meet eligibility requirements. If the patient is impoverished, he or she may then qualify for Medicaid, which will cover long-term care expenses. Medicaid pays for almost half of all nursing home care in the United States; patients and their families pay for the rest. For those who can afford it, long-term care insurance can cover expenses beyond 100 days.

It is difficult to predict who will need long-term care insurance. One percent of individuals between the ages of 65 and 74 reside in a nursing home, while 7% of those between 75 and 84, and more than 20% of those age 85 or older reside in nursing homes. Long-term care insurance is relatively new, and there are a variety of plans and benefits available. These policies can be expensive and, while an average policy costs only $2000 per year for people in their early 60s, premiums rise to more than $7000 per year for those over age 75. Average long-term care costs are detailed below.

| Type of Care | Cost |
| --- | --- |
| Skilled nursing facility | $45,000/year |
| Intermediate care facility | $40,000/year |
| Custodial care facility | $36,000/year |
| Home care attendant | $15/hour |

*Skilled nursing home care* is the highest level of care provided. This is for individuals who require intensive 24-hour care provided by skilled, licensed professionals such as registered nurses or physical therapists. Care is usually provided to complete medical treatment or to provide intensive rehabilitation.

An *intermediate nursing care* facility is similar to a skilled-care facility but provides care for stable conditions that require daily, but not 24-hour, nursing supervision. It often involves more personal care and is generally needed for a longer period of time.

A *custodial care* facility furnishes the patient with help for activities of daily living (ADL) such as eating, bathing, dressing, and moving about. This care is provided by people without medical skills. Custodial care can be provided in many settings, including nursing homes, adult day centers, respite centers, or at home.

*Home care* is administered in a person's home and may include part-time skilled nursing care, physical or occupational therapy, or a home health aide.

# CHAPTER 6

# PHARMACEUTICAL COSTS

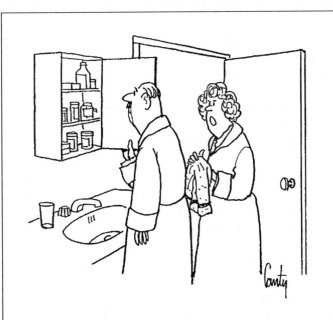

*"Just take your medication and don't concern yourself with its street value."*

**P**rescription medications are an area of rapidly escalating costs. Over the last decade, there has been an explosion in the creation of pharmaceutical agents, many of which have been helpful in treating a variety of patient problems. However, in addition to the development of new drug classes, we have been introduced to numerous new brands of medications within the same classes. Although we might think that such competition would help control costs, this has not been the case. Frequently, when a company produces a "copycat" drug, the price is even higher than the one already on the market.

In order to sell their drugs, pharmaceutical representatives market directly to physicians using a practice known as "detailing." The pharmaceutical representative visits individual physicians and tries to convince them to prescribe their company's products over other available brands. Many physicians are concerned about this practice, as this is a direct sales technique and representatives may not always be up-front (or objective) about the best medication to use for patients. Indeed, some insurance companies, like Blue Cross's Optimal Therapeutic Program, attempt to counter the advertising and drug-detailing done by the pharmaceutical companies. Representatives from the insurance company (often a pharmacist) will visit physician offices to discuss appropriate medication choices and how to prescribe in a cost-effective manner. Some of the drug-cost lists in this chapter were provided by the Optimal program.

In an attempt to control rising drug costs, several measures have been instituted. Most states have passed legislation allowing pharmacies to fill prescriptions written by physicians with generic equivalents. This occurs even if the physician has prescribed a name brand. In order to have the particular brand dispensed, the physician must specifically write the brand name and add a statement like "no substitution" on the prescription. A *generic equivalent* is a less expensive medication equivalent to the commonly known brand name. There has been some debate about the safety of generics, but the U.S. Food and Drug Administration (FDA) has recently tightened safety regulations on generic medications, and many brand name companies now manufacture generic equivalents.

Formularies have been developed in an attempt to control drug costs. A *formulary* is a restrictive list of available medications from which physicians must choose. Hospitals have used formularies for a number of years. Traditionally, a hospital formulary would include a few brands of medications for any given class of drug. The physician was "restricted" in that only medications from this list could be ordered for his or her patients. Since the advent of diagnosis-related groups (DRGs), hospital pharmacies have been more aggressive about limiting their formularies. Cost of the medication, rather than physician preference, is a principal factor in determining which drugs to include in the formulary.

In the outpatient setting, health maintenance organizations (HMOs), preferred provider organizations (PPOs), and individual practice associations (IPAs) are also beginning to restrict physician prescribing practices. This is accomplished through a formulary process, much like the hospital formularies. A recent survey indicated that more than 70% of HMOs are moving toward formularies for their patients (Figure 6.1). Some plans are quite restrictive, whereas others allow physicians more choice, while attempting to educate them about the costs associated with their prescriptions. Typically, the managed care organization (MCO) will provide the physician with a small notebook that lists the covered medications and their comparative costs. This helps the physician to prescribe lower-cost alternatives. Table 6.1 illustrates how such a formulary is commonly organized.

While the physicians are free to prescribe any medication from the formulary, they are often encouraged (via cost incentives) to prescribe low-cost formulary alternatives. Both "carrot" and "stick" incentives are used. *Carrot*

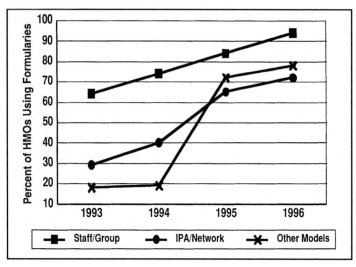

**Figure 6.1** *Percent of HMOs using formularies, 1993–1996. (IPA = individual practice association.)*

*incentives* reward physicians who prescribe low-cost formulary choices by paying bonuses at the end of the year if the plan's pharmaceutical costs are under budget. *Stick incentives* are just the opposite, with the physician being financially penalized if the plan's pharmaceutical budget has been overspent.

Patients also put pressure on their physicians to prescribe drugs from the formulary, because patients must pay for medications if they are themselves not covered by their insurance.

The following pages outline how varied prices are for medications with essentially the same indications (Figures 6.2, 6.3; Tables 6.2–6.8). Take a few minutes to review these charts and tables. Become familiar with the less expensive alternatives and incorporate them into your prescribing patterns. Physicians can learn more about drug costs by subscribing to *The Medical Letter* (1-800-211-2769). This nonprofit publication reviews newly-released medications and periodically reviews the expense profiles for classes of drugs. Some tables from *The Medical Letter* are included here.

*Note:* A word of caution about using these medication price lists—pricing is fluid. Prices of brand-name products usually drop when generic equivalents become available; however, they may also rise. Moreover, any given MCO can contract with a pharmaceutical company for a large discount for a particular drug. One strategy to consider might be to prescribe generic drugs, thereby obviating the need to remember what brand is on which formulary. Thus, while the attached prices given in the following tables can be used as guidelines, they are not definitive prices and may vary for different regions of the United States. If you cannot locate your drug of choice in the tables, call your local pharmacist for prices.

## A PAGE FROM A DRUG FORMULARY

**ACE Inhibitors***  $8–$60

Guidelines for the treatment of hypertension recommend the use of ACE inhibitors as alternative agents for initial monotherapy. Quinapril (Accupril), lisinopril (Zestril), captopril (Capoten), and enalapril (Vasotec) are indicated for hypertension and congestive heart failure. Enalapril offers no significant benefit (clinical/cost) over the ACE inhibitors and is a nonformulary agent.

Captopril, indicated for the treatment of diabetic nephropathy, has been proven to slow the progression of diabetic kidney disease.

| | | | |
|---|---|---|---|
| quinapril | Accupril | $ | (preferred) |
| benazepril | Lotensin | $$ | |
| fosinopril | Monopril | $$ | |
| lisinopril | Zestril | $$ | |
| ramipril | Altace | $$ | |
| enalapril | Vasotec (NF) | $$$ | |
| captopril | Capoten | $$$$ | |

■ Table 6.1
*NF = nonformulary; $ = least expensive; $$$$ = most expensive.*

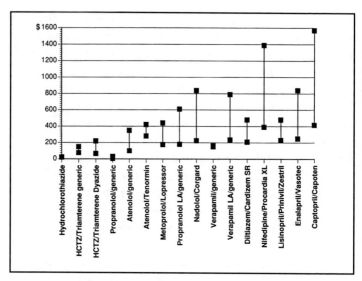

**Figure 6.2** *Costs of blood-pressure lowering medications. (Costs calculated in 1994 and based on one year of use; HCTZ =
hydrochlorothiazide.)*

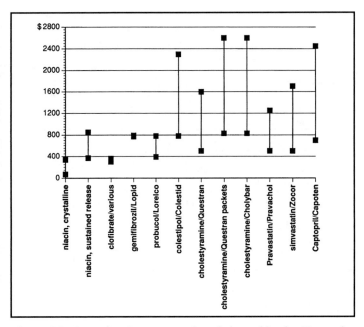

**Figure 6.3** *Costs of medications to reduce cholesterol levels. (Costs calculated in 1994 and based on one year of use.)*

## RETAIL PRICES FOR COMMON
## OVER-THE-COUNTER MEDICATIONS

| Medication | Quantity | Brand ($) | Generic ($) |
|---|---|---|---|
| Chlor-Trimeton (chlorpheniramine maleate) | 4 mg #24 | 4.58 | 2.76[a] |
| Benadryl (diphenhydramine) | 25 mg #24 | 3.42 | 1.97 |
| Dimetapp | #12 | 4.37 | 1.97 |
| Sudafed (pseudoephedrine) | 30 mg #24 | 3.27 | 1.31 |
| Robitussin DM (dextro-methorphan/guaifenesin) | #4 oz | 3.87 | 1.66 |
| Advil (ibuprofen) | 200 mg #50 | 4.56 | 1.96 |
| Aspirin (Bayer) | 325 mg #100 | 4.46 | 2.37[b] |
| Tylenol (acetaminophen) | 325.mg #100 | 6.96 | 3.27 |
| Kaopectate (kaolin/pectin) | #8 oz | 3.94 | N/A |
| Mylicon (simethicone) | 80 mg #100 | 11.37 | N/A |
| Mylanta II (simethicone/antacid) | #12 oz | 4.54 | 2.26 |
| Dulcolax (bisacodyl) | Supp #8 | 6.97 | 2.97 |
| Colace (docusate sodium) | 100 mg #30 | 8.32 | 1.97 |
| Anusol (bismuth subgallate) | Supp #12 | 5.17 | N/A |
| Metamucil (psyllium seed mucilloid) | #21 oz | 9.87 | 4.27 |
| Senokot (senna fruit) | #100 | 16.56 | 12.99 |
| Neosporin (neomycin/poly-myxin B/bacitracin | #1 oz | 5.56 | 2.57 |
| Debrox (carbamide peroxide) | #0.5 oz | 5.38 | 2.97 |
| Tagamet | #12 | 4.87 | N/A |
| Zantac | #30 | 8.17 | N/A |
| Pepcid AC | #30 | 7.97 | N/A |
| Minoxidil (rogaine) | #60 cc | 12.97 | N/A |

■ Table 6.2

*N/A = not available.*
[a] *Generic Chlor-trimeton: 100 tabs/2.76.*
[b] *Generic aspirin: 300 tabs/2.37.*

## RETAIL PRICES FOR SELECTED PRESCRIPTION MEDICATIONS

| Antibiotics | Quantity | Price ($) |
|---|---|---|
| Ketoconazole (Nizoral) | 200 mg #30 | 92.78* |
| Griseofulvin (Fulvicin-U/F) | 500 mg #30 | 45.62* |
| Sporonox | 100 mg #30 | 179.97* |
| Lamisil | 250 mg #30 | 192.46* |
| Cefaclor (Ceclor) | 250 mg/5 ml #150 cc | 50.78* |
| Erythromycin (Ery-tab) | 333 mg #30 | 8.46* |
| EES (erythromycin ethylsuccinate) | 200 mg/5 ml #200 cc | 10.72 |
| Biaxin | 500 mg #20 | 64.46* |
| Zithromax | 250 mg #6 | 38.84* |
| Amoxicillin | 125 mg/5 ml #150 cc<br>250 mg/5 ml #150 cc<br>250 mg #30 | 7.68<br>8.97<br>6.98 |
| Amoxicillin/clavulanic acid (Augmentin) | 125 mg/5 ml #150 cc<br>250 mg/5 ml #150 cc<br>250 mg #30 | 34.97*<br>62.54*<br>65.98* |
| Dicloxacillin (Dynapen) | 250 mg #30 | 10.46 |
| Doxycycline hyclate (Vibramycin) | 50 mg #20 | 10.68 |
| Tetracycline | 250 mg #40 | 6.54 |
| Cephalexin monohydrate (Keflex) | 250 mg #40 | 13.92 |
| Cefixime (Suprax) | 100 mg/5 ml #100 cc | 68.92 |
| Ciprofloxacin (Cipro) | 250 mg #40 | 122.20* |
| Norfloxacin (Noroxin) | 400 mg #20 | 62.32* |
| Nitrofurantoin (Macrodantin) | 100 mg #40 | 31.46 |
| Co-trimaxazole (Bactrim DS) | #20 | 10.46 |
| **Antiviral** | | |
| Acyclovir (Zovirax) | 200 mg #50<br>800 mg #30 | 40.68<br>75.92 |
| Amantadine (Symmetrel) | 200 mg #30 | 13.78 |
| Zidovudine (AZT) | 100 mg #150 | 241.97* |

■ **Table 6.3**
*Brand-name price.*

| Seizure Medications | Quantity | Price ($) |
|---|---|---|
| Phenobarbital | 60 mg #100 | 7.54 |
| Phenytoin (Dilantin) | 100 mg #100 | 23.92* |
| Carbamazepine (Tegretol) | 200 mg #100 | 20.78 |
| **Antidepressants/Anxiolytics** | | |
| Amitriptyline (Elavil) | 50 mg #100 | 9.92 |
| Doxepin (Sinequan) | 50 mg #100 | 15.72 |
| Imipramine (Tofranil) | 50 mg #100 | 11.84 |
| Trazodone (Desyrel) | 50 mg #90 | 12.79 |
| Alprazolam (Xanax) | 0.25 mg #30 | 9.84 |
| Diazepam (Valium) | 5 mg #30 | 6.78 |
| Lorazepam (Ativan) | 2 mg #30 | 7.72 |
| Prozac | 20 mg #30 | 68.29* |
| Zoloft | 50 mg #30 | 56.98* |
| **Asthma/COPD Medications** | | |
| Albuterol (Proventil, Ventolin) | Inhaler | 16.98 |
| Metaproterenol (Alupent, Metaprel) | Inhaler | 24.68* |
| Cromolyn (Intal) 8.1 gm | Inhaler | 42.78* |
| Triamcinolone (Azmacort) | Inhaler | 44.97* |
| Ipratropium bromide (Atrovent) | Inhaler | 29.97* |
| Beclomethasone dipropionate (Vanceril) | Inhaler | 35.78* |
| Theophylline (Theodur) | 200 mg #90 | 17.68 |
| **Ulcer Medications** | | |
| Ranitidine (Zantac) | 150 mg #30 | 45.84* |
| Cimetidine (Tagamet) | 300 mg #30 | 16.46 |
| Sucralfate (Carafate) | 1 gm #100 | 60.72 |
| Omeprazole (Prilosec) | 20 mg #30 | 99.97* |
| Misoprostol (Cytotec) | 200 μg #100 | 77.62* |

■ **Table 6.3** *(continued)*
*COPD = chronic obstructive pulmonary disease.*
*\*Brand-name price.*

| Diabetes Medications | Quantity | Price ($) |
|---|---|---|
| Chlorpropamide (Diabinese) | 250 mg #100 | 16.72 |
| Tolbutamide (Orinase) | 250 mg #30 | 6.92 |
| Glipizide (Glucotrol) | 10 mg #30 | 16.46 |
| Insulin | | |
|   Regular | #10 ml/bottle | 15.98* |
|   NPH | #10 ml/bottle | 15.98* |
|   Humulin | #10 ml/bottle | 16.93* |
| **Cholesterol Medications** | | |
| Cholestyramine (Questran) | Pkg #30 | 26.46 |
| Lovastatin (Mevacor) | 20 mg #30 | 57.65* |
| Gemfibrozil (Lopid) | 600 mg #60 | 23.62 |
| Zocor (Simvastatin) | 20 mg #30 | 95.72* |
| **Oral Estrogens** | | |
| Brevicon | Pkg | 23.78* |
| Lo/Ovral | Pkg | 23.22* |
| Ortho Novum 1/35 | Pkg | 9.98 |
| Triphasil | Pkg | 21.78 |
| Estrogen (Premarin) | 0.625 mg #30 | 11.98* |
| **Miscellaneous Medications** | | |
| Sodium fluoride (Luride) | 1 mg #120 | 4.55 |
| Levothyroxine (Synthroid) | 0.1 mg #30 | 5.64 |
| Ergotamine tartrate (Cafergot) | #20 | 20.46 |
| Ferrous sulfate | 325 mg #100 | 1.67 |
| Warfarin sodium (Coumadin) | 5 mg #30 | 19.71* |
| Cyclobenzaprine hydrochloride (Flexeril) | 10 mg #30 | 13.78 |
| Lindane (Kwell) | Shampoo #2 oz | 8.62 |
| Prednisone (Orasone) | 20 mg #20 | 6.72 |
| Terfenadine (Seldane) | 60 mg #30 | 29.54 |

■ **Table 6.3** *(continued)*
*Brand-name price.*

| Miscellaneous Medications (cont.) | Quantity | Price ($) |
|---|---|---|
| Claritin | 10 mg #30 | 60.62* |
| Hismanal | 10 mg #30 | 57.98* |
| Diphenoxylate/atropine (Lomotil) | #30 | 7.72 |
| Prochlorperazine (Compazine) | 25 mg, Supp #12 | 30.97 |
| **Cardiac Medications** | | |
| Atenolol (Tenormin) | 50 mg #30 | 4.98 |
| Digoxin (Lanoxin) | 0.25 mg #30 | 5.84 |
| Diltiazem (Cardizem) | 60 mg #120 | 23.19 |
| Enalapril (Vasotec) | 10 mg #30 | 27.98* |
| Metoprolol (Lopressor) | 50 mg #30 | 4.73 |
| Nifedipine (Procardia XL) | 30 mg #30 | 37.06 |
| Procainamide (Pronestyl) | 375 mg #90 | 9.78 |
| Propranolol (Inderal) (LA) | 40 mg #100<br>160 mg #30 | 13.78<br>35.62 |
| Verapamil (Calan SR) | 240 mg #30 | 24.84 |
| Captopril (Capoten) | 25 mg #90 | 26.54 |
| Clonidine (Catapres) (0.1) | 0.1 mg #60<br>Patch #4 | 7.98<br>35.78* |
| Hydralazine (Apresoline) | 10 mg #120 | 7.97 |
| Dipyridamole (Persantine) | 75 mg #100 | 8.97 |
| Isosorbide Dinitrate (Isordil) | 10 mg #120 | 8.78 |
| Nitroglycerin SL (Nitrostat) | 0.4 mg #100 | 9.54* |
| Bumetanide (Bumex) | 0.5 mg #30 | 13.78 |
| Hydrochlorothiazide (Esidrix) | 25 mg #30 | 2.97 |
| Furosemide (Lasix) | 40 mg #100 | 5.98 |
| Spironolactone (Aldactone) | 25 mg #30 | 9.84 |
| Potassium chloride (Micro-K) | 10 mEq #30 | 8.78 |

■ **Table 6.3** *(continued)*
*Brand-name price.*

| NSAIDs | Quantity | Price ($) |
|---|---|---|
| Indomethacin (Indocin) | 25 mg #60 | 13.78 |
| Naproxen (Naprosyn) | 375 mg #40 | 14.92 |
| Salsalate (Disalcid) | 500 mg #40 | 9.78 |
| Sulindac (Clinoril) | 150 mg #40 | 16.97 |
| Ketoprofen (Orudis)<br>(Generic) | 50 mg #30<br>50 mg #30 | 27.87<br>14.46 |
| Ibuprofen (Motrin) | 600 mg #100 | 8.97 |
| Diflunisal (Dolobid) | 500 mg #20 | 19.62 |
| **Pain Medications** | | |
| Codeine/acetaminophen<br>(Tylenol No. 3) | #20 | 6.72 |
| Meperidine (Demerol) | 50 mg #20 | 11.54 |
| Oxycodone/acetaminophen<br>(Percocet) | #20 | 12.46 |
| Fiorinal | #20 | 7.54 |

■ **Table 6.3** *(continued)*
*NSAIDs = nonsteroidal anti-inflammatory drugs.*
*\*Brand-name price.*

## Cost of Some Lipid-Lowering Drugs

| Drug | Daily Dosage | Cost[a] |
|------|--------------|------|
| Atorvastatin (*Lipitor* – Parke-Davis) | 10 mg once | $ 54.72 |
| Fluvastatin (*Lescol* – Novartis) | 20 mg once[b] | 36.60 |
| Lovastatin (*Mevacor* – Merck) | 20 mg once | 67.50 |
| Pravastatin (*Pravachol* – Bristol-Myers Squibb) | 20 mg once | 58.97 |
| Simvastatin (*Zocor* – Merck) | 10 mg once | 60.86 |
| Cholestyramine – average generic price (*Questran, Questran Light* – Bristol-Myers Squibb) (*Prevalite* packets – Upsher-Smith) | 8 gm resin, divided | 50.31 55.90 59.80 |
| Colestipol (*Colestid* – Pharmacia & Upjohn) (*Colestid* tablets) | 10 gm, divided 10 gm, divided | 51.43 94.90 |
| Clofibrate (*Atromid S* – Wyeth-Ayerst) | 1 gm bid | 106.50 |
| Gemfibrozil (*Lopid* – Parke-Davis) | 600 mg bid | 75.23 |
| Niacin – generic price (*Niacor* – Upsher-Smith) (*Nicolar* – Rhône-Poulenc Rorer) | 1 gm tid | 5.38 27.79 121.72 |

■ **Table 6.4**

[a] *Cost to the pharmacist for 30 days' treatment based on wholesale price (AWP or HCFA) listings in* Drug Topics Red Book 1996 and March 1997 Update.

[b] *Dosage recommended by manufacturer, but appears to be less effective than recommended doses of atorvastatin, lovastatin, pravastatin, and simvastatin.*

*Source: Atrovastatin—A new lipid-lowering drug.* Med Lett Drugs Ther 1997;39:29.

## Cost of Some Psychiatric Drugs

| Drug | Usual Daily Dosage | Cost[a] |
|---|---|---|
| **Antidepressant Drugs** | | |
| Amitriptyline – generic price (*Elavil* – Zeneca) | 200 mg once/day | $ 2.57 74.48 |
| Bupropion (*Wellbutrin* – Glaxo Wellcome) (*Wellbutrin* SR) | 100 mg tid 150 mg bid | 74.66 73.70 |
| Desipramine – generic price (*Norpramin* – Hoechst Marion Roussel) | 200 mg once/day | 24.53 114.34 |
| Fluoxetine (*Prozac* – Dista) | 20 mg once/day | 72.51 |
| Imipramine – generic price (*Tofranil PM* – Novartis) | 200 mg once/day | 3.70 88.02 |
| Mirtazapine (*Remeron* – Organon) | 30 mg once/day | 61.20 |
| Nefazodone (*Serzone* – Bristol-Myers Squibb) | 200 mg bid | 58.14 |
| Nortriptyline – generic price (*Pamelor* – Novartis) | 100 mg once/day | 11.66 118.58 |
| Paroxetine (*Paxil* – SmithKline Beecham) | 20 mg once/day | 61.95 |
| Phenelzine (*Nardil* – Parke-Davis) | 30 mg bid | 48.29 |
| Sertraline (*Zoloft* – Roerig) | 100 mg once/day | 66.54 |
| Trazodone – generic price (*Desyrel* – Apothecon) (*Desyrel Dividose*) | 300 mg in divided doses | 10.53 230.47 104.47 |
| Venlafaxine (*Effexor* – Wyeth-Ayerst) | 75 mg bid | 68.68 |
| **Drugs for Anxiety** | | |
| Alprazolam (*Xanax* – Pharmacia & Upjohn) | 0.5 mg qid[b] | 97.43 |
| Clonazepam – generic price (*Klonopin* – Roche) | 0.5 mg bid[b] | 42.46 48.14 |

■ Table 6.5

| Drug | Usual Daily Dosage | Cost[a] |
|------|--------------------|---------|
| **Drugs for Anxiety** *(cont.)* | | |
| Diazepam – generic price (*Valium* – Roche) | 10 mg bid | 1.48 66.65 |
| Lorazepam – generic price (*Ativan* – Wyeth-Ayerst) | 1 mg tid | 1.86 80.24 |
| Oxazepam – generic price (*Serax* – Wyeth-Ayerst) | 15 mg tid | 6.35 86.90 |
| Buspirone (*Buspar* – Bristol-Myers Squibb) | 15 mg bid | 101.09 |
| **Drugs for OCD** | | |
| Clomipramine (*Anafranil* – Novartis) | 200 mg once/day | 129.89 |
| Fluvoxamine (*Luvox* – Solvay) | 100 mg bid | 127.53 |
| **Drugs for Mania** | | |
| Carbamazepine – generic price (*Tegretol-XR* – Novartis) | 400 mg bid | 17.60 47.70 |
| Divalproex sodium (*Depakote* – Abbott) | 750 mg bid | 109.48 |
| Lithium – generic price | 1500 mg/day in divided doses | 7.88 |
| (*Eskalith* – SmithKline Beecham) (*Lithobid* – Solvay) (*Lithonate* – Solvay) | | 27.83 39.60 12.60 |

■ **Table 6.5** *(continued)*

*OCD = obsessive-compulsive disorder.*

[a] *Cost to the pharmacist for a 30-day supply based on wholesale price (AWP or HCFA) listings in* Drug Topics Red Book *1996 and March 1997* Update.

[b] *Patients with panic disorder often require higher dosage.*

*Source: Drugs for psychiatric disorders.* Med Lett Drugs Ther *1997;39:36.*

## Cost of Angiotensin II Receptor Antagonists and ACE Inhibitors for Hypertension

| Drug | Daily Dosage | Cost* |
|---|---|---|
| **Angiotensin II Receptor Antagonists** | | |
| Losartan (*Cozaar* – Merck) | Initial: 50 mg once<br>Usual: 25–100 mg<br>once or divided | $ 35.10 |
| Valsartan (*Diovan* – Novartis) | Initial: 80 mg once<br>Usual: 80–320 mg<br>once | 34.21 |
| **ACE Inhibitors** | | |
| Benazepril (*Lotensin* – Novartis) | Initial: 10 mg once<br>Usual: 20–40 mg<br>once or divided | 20.84 |
| Captopril – generic price<br><br>(*Capoten* – Bristol-Myers Squibb) | Initial: 25 mg<br>bid or tid<br>Usual: 25–150 mg<br>bid or tid | 4.00<br><br>47.06 |
| Enalapril (*Vasotec* – Merck) | Initial: 5 mg once<br>Usual: 10–40 mg<br>once or divided | 30.88 |
| Fosinopril (*Monopril* – Bristol-Myers Squibb) | Initial: 10 mg once<br>Usual: 20–40 mg<br>once or bid | 23.92 |
| Lisinopril (*Prinivil* – Merck)<br>(*Zestril* – Stuart) | Initial: 10 mg once<br>Usual: 20–40 mg<br>once | 27.11<br>27.14 |

■ **Table 6.6**

*ACE = angiotensin-converting enzyme.*
*\*Cost to the pharmacist for 30 days' treatment with the lowest usual dosage, according to wholesale price (AWP or HCFA) listings in* Drug Topics Red Book Update, *April 1997.*
*Source: Valsartan for hypertension.* Med Lett Drugs Ther *1997;39:44.*

| ACE Inhibitors *(cont.)* | | |
|---|---|---|
| Moexipril (*Univasc* – Schwarz) | Initial: 7.5 mg once<br>Usual: 7.5–30 mg<br>once or divided | 14.91 |
| Quinapril (*Accupril* – Parke-Davis) | Initial: 10 mg once<br>Usual: 20–80 mg<br>once or divided | 28.50 |
| Ramipril (*Altace* – Hoechst Marion Roussel) | Initial: 2.5 mg once<br>Usual: 2.5–20 mg<br>once or divided | 22.66 |
| Trandolapril (*Mavik* – Knoll) | Initial: 1 or 2 mg<br>once<br>Usual: 2–4 mg once | 18.00 |

■ **Table 6.6** *(continued)*

## COST OF SOME TOPICAL DRUGS FOR ACNE

| Drug | Formulation[a] | Cost[b] |
|---|---|---|
| Adapalene <br> (*Differin* – Galderma) | 0.1% gel | 15 gm –   $22.08 |
| Antibiotics <br>   Clindamycin <br>     (*CleocinT* – Upjohn) | 1% gel (solution, lotion) | 30 gm –    22.04 |
|   Erythromycin <br>     (*Emgel* – Glaxo Wellcome) <br>     (*Erycette* – Ortho) <br>     (*T-Stat*-Westwood-Squibb) | 2% gel <br> 2% solution <br> 2% solution | 27 gm –    18.97 <br> 60 swabs – 21.24 <br> 60 ml –    17.21 <br> 60 pads –   19.33 |
|   Erythromycin/benzoyl peroxide <br>     (*Benzamycin* – Dermik) | 3%/5% gel | 23.3 gm –  29.99 |
| Azelaic acid (*Azelex* – Allergan) | 20% cream | 30 gm –    28.88 |
| Benzoyl peroxide[c] <br>   average generic price | 5% gel <br> 10% gel | 45 gm –     1.99 <br> 45 gm –     2.22 |
| Tretinoin <br>   (*Retin-A* – Ortho) | 0.01% gel <br> 0.025% gel <br> 0.025% cream <br> 0.05% cream <br> 0.1% cream <br> 0.05% liquid | 15 gm –    22.74 <br> 15 gm –    22.98 <br> 20 gm –    28.20 <br> 20 gm –    29.28 <br> 20 gm –    34.14 <br> 28 ml –    44.94 |

■ **Table 6.7**

[a] *Other available formulations are listed in parentheses.*

[b] *Cost to the pharmacist for the smallest size available, based on wholesale price (AWP) listings in* Drug Topics Red Book 1996 *and* Microdata Plus, *February 1997.*

[c] *Available without a prescription.*

*Source: Adapalene for acne. Med Lett Drugs Ther 1997;39:20.*

## COST OF SOME NONSTEROIDAL
## ANTI-INFLAMMATORY DRUGS

| Drug | Usual Dosage Range for Arthritis | Cost[a] |
|---|---|---|
| Aspirin, extended-release – average generic price (range: $9.64 to $15.42) (*Extended Release Bayer 8 Hour*[b] – Sterling) (*ZORprin* – Boots) | 1600 mg bid<br><br>1300 mg tid<br><br>1600 mg to 3200 mg bid | $  12.65<br><br>17.25<br><br>34.86 |
| Aspirin, enteric-coated[b] – average generic price (range: $3.24 to $12.00) (*Extra Strength Bayer Enteric Aspirin*[b]) | 1000 mg qid | 7.14<br><br>28.42 |
| Non-acetylated salicylates<br> Magnesium salicylate (*Magan* – Savage)<br> Choline salicylate (*Arthropan* – Purdue Frederick)<br> Choline magnesium salicylate – average generic price (range: $40.32 to $60.08) | 1090 mg tid–qid<br><br>4.8 to 7.2 gm/day divided<br><br>3 gm/day in 1, 2, or 3 doses | 82.71<br><br>54.77<br><br>47.16 |

■ **Table 6.8**

[a] *Cost to the pharmacist for 30 days' treatment with the lowest usual dosage, based on wholesale price (AWP) listings in* Red Book 1994 *and* October Update.

[b] *Available without a prescription.*

[c] *Also available as liquid formulation.*

[d] *Also available without prescription in a lower tablet strength.*

*Source: Drugs for rheumatoid arthritis.* Med Lett Drugs Ther *1994;36:102.*

| Drug | Usual Dosage Range for Arthritis | Cost[a] |
|------|----------------------------------|---------|
| (*Trilisate* – Purdue Frederick)[c] | | 81.21 |
| Sodium salicylate[b] – average generic price (range: $2.79 to $6.45) | 3.6 to 5.4 gm/day divided doses | 4.35 |
| Salicylsalicylic acid (salsalate) – average generic price (range: $13.72 to $54.32) | 3 to 4 gm/day in 2 or 3 doses | 27.95 |
| (*Disalcid* – 3M) | | 55.66 |
| (*Mono-Gesic* – Central) | | 33.42 |
| Diclofenac (*Voltaren* – Ciba-Geigy) | 150 to 200 mg/day in 2 or 3 doses | 66.23 |
| Diflunisal – average generic price (range: $23.33 to $30.12) | 500 to 1000 mg/day in 2 doses | 28.54 |
| (*Dolobid* – MSD) | | 34.57 |
| Fenoprofen – average generic price (range: $24.63 to $31.94) | 300 to 600 mg tid–qid | 29.75 |
| (*Nalfon* – Dista) | | 34.88 |
| Flurbiprofen (*Ansaid* – Upjohn) | 200 to 300 mg/day in 2, 3, or 4 doses | 71.72 |
| Ibuprofen[d] – average generic price (range: $5.09 to $14.36) | 1200 to 3200 mg/day in 3 or 4 doses | 9.51 |
| (*Motrin* – Upjohn) | | 17.85 |
| (*Rufen* – Boots) | | 16.56 |

■ **Table 6.8** (*continued*)

| Drug | Usual Dosage Range for Arthritis | Cost[a] |
|------|----------------------------------|---------|
| Indomethacin – average generic price (range: $4.91 to $22.10) | 25 to 50 mg tid–qid | 10.38 |
| (*Indocin* – MSD) extended-release– average generic price (range: $27.50 to $36.38) | 75 mg once/day or bid | 46.99<br>30.95 |
| (*Indocin SR* – MSD) | | 42.13 |
| Ketoprofen – average generic price (range: $72.56 to $80.33) | 50 to 75 mg tid–qid | 77.70 |
| (*Orudis* – Wyeth-Ayerst) | | 89.11 |
| (*Oruvail* – Wyeth-Ayerst) | 200 mg once/day | 62.07 |
| Meclofenamate sodium – average generic price (range: $20.40 to $61.20) | 200 to 400 mg/day in 3 or 4 doses | 40.62 |
| (*Meclomen* – Parke-Davis) | | 88.94 |
| Nabumetone (*Relafen* – SmithKline Beecham) | 1000 once/day to 2000 mg day | 58.68 |
| Naproxen – average generic price (range $39.80 to $45.73) | 250 to 500 mg bid–tid | 41.05 |
| (*Naprosyn* – Syntex)[c] | | 46.46 |
| Naproxen sodium[d] – average generic price (range: $36.00 to $41.01) | 275 mg or 550 mg bid | 39.79 |
| (*Anaprox* – Syntex) | | 46.31 |

■ **Table 6.8** *(continued)*

| Drug | Usual Dosage Range for Arthritis | Cost[a] |
|------|----------------------------------|---------|
| Oxaprozin (*Daypro* – Searle) | 1200 mg once/day to 1800 mg | 70.01 |
| Piroxicam – average generic price (range: $39.00 to $67.67) (*Feldene* – Pfizer) | 20 mg once/day | 60.90 <br><br> 74.21 |
| Sulindac – average generic price (range: $31.82 to $50.55) (*Clinoril* – MSD) | 150 to 200 mg bid | 45.51 <br><br> 55.95 |
| Tolmetin – average generic price (range: $31.03 to $36.45) (*Tolectin* – McNeil) | 600 to 1800 mg/day in 3 or 4 doses | 34.20 <br><br> 54.96 |

■ **Table 6.8** (*continued*)

# CHAPTER 7

# PROBLEM-SOLVING EXERCISES

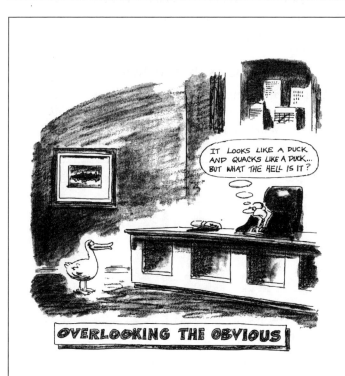

# MANAGED CARE EXERCISE

**M**anaged care has become an integral part of medicine. Managed care systems affect physicians, regardless of specialty choice. In primary care practices, physicians typically contract with a number of managed care organizations. The primary care physician acts as the patient's primary physician and arranges care as appropriate. Managed care plans typically affect primary care physicians by requiring the use of selected specialty referrals, pharmaceutical formularies, and utilization review of inpatient practices. Additionally, there are restrictions regarding payment, from discounted fees and withholds, to capitated payment plans. You can learn a lot about managed care by answering the following questions with the help of a primary care preceptor.

## A—The Physician's Perspective

1. List two managed care plans that your preceptor participates in and categorize them (i.e., HMO, PPO, etc.). What do these terms mean?

   **Plan Name:** _____

   **Type:** _____

   **Define:** _____

   **Plan Name:** _____

   **Type:** _____

   **Define:** _____

**2.** Are there any pharmaceutical prescribing restrictions placed on your preceptor, such as the use of formularies? What observations do you have about these formularies and how they impact on your preceptor's practice? How will you incorporate the use of such formularies into your future practice?

**3.** How are subspecialty referrals obtained? Are there restrictions regarding who can be used as a referral source? Are there particular forms? How has your preceptor changed his or her practice in order to deal with requirements for referrals in managed care plans?

**4.** Part of managed care is keeping patients out of emergency rooms and hospitals. Comment on any particular problems that your preceptor has had in this regard and what he or she has done to incorporate utilization review practices into the care of inpatients.

5. Does your preceptor participate in capitated payment plans? If so, give a brief review of how this capitation works (i.e., amount/member/monthly payment for ancillary services) and how your preceptor perceives its impact on his or her practice.

6. Many managed care plans withhold partial payments and only pay the physician if the plan has a profit at the end of the year. Identify problems that your preceptor has encountered with withholds, and how he or she has coped with them.

## B—The Patient's Perspective

Identify a patient to discuss how he or she pays for health care. Answer the following questions:

1. What type of insurance does the patient have?

_____ **HMO**

_____ **IPA**

_____ **PPO**

_____ **Indemnity**

_____ **Government sponsored**

_____ **Other**

_____ **None** (If the patient does not have any health insurance, how does he or she pay for health care? What resources has the patient explored in attempting to obtain insurance?)

2. How has the patient obtained this insurance?

_____ **Through employer or spouse's employer**

_____ **Pays for by self**

_____ **Governmental program** (Medicaid) (Explore how the patient received this coverage and what he or she needs to do to stay in the program.)

3. Cost of insurance for this patient's family:

$_____ **Total cost**

$_____ **Payroll deduction (patient portion)**

$_____ **Direct payments**

$_____ **Deductibles**

$_____ **Other**

**4.** How does the patient pay for medications?

_____ **Out of pocket**
_____ **Copayment of $_____ for 1-month supply**
_____ **Medicaid patient**
_____ **Meets deductible**

**5.** Are there any services that the patient needs or wants that his or her insurance does not cover?  Explain.

**6.** Determine the patient's general level of satisfaction with his or her insurance.  Explain.

**7.** Fill out the following table for any health-care expenses encountered by this patient for illnesses this year.

| | Actual Cost | Patient Payment | Insurance Coverage |
|---|---|---|---|
| Medications (prescription and over-the-counter) | | | |
| Supplies/appliances (e.g., oxygen, syringes, etc.) | | | |
| Services (nursing, physical therapy, etc.) | | | |
| Other costs (transportation, days out of work, etc.) | | | |
| Physician charges | | | |
| Laboratory/ examination charges | | | |
| Hospital charges | | | |
| Total cost of illness | | | |

# PROBLEM-SOLVING CASES

When deciding on a diagnostic workup for your patients, consider the costs of laboratory, radiologic, and other diagnostic techniques. Although it is not necessary to know what the exact charges are, it is important to have a sense of the cost and to understand that less expensive alternatives may provide sufficient information for your needs.

In addition to careful consideration of the workup, it is important to avoid the "shotgun" approach. Before ordering any diagnostic test, ask yourself, "Will this change my diagnosis or therapy?" If you have already decided on a treatment plan based on the patient's history and results of the physical examination, it is not always necessary to pursue ancillary testing merely to confirm or "rule-out" other conditions. Rely on your clinical skills and understand the importance of two concepts: continuity of care, and patient centered care. Discuss your thoughts with the patient, plan for the patient to return at an appropriate interval, and reconsider your diagnostic and treatment workup if necessary.

The following cases will begin to familiarize you with the costs associated with a variety of common diagnostic and treatment modalities. As you work through each case, choose your options thoughtfully and estimate the cost of your care. Fill in your choice before looking in Appendix A for the answers—you may be surprised at the differences. The answers are explained and, although they may differ from what you would do, it does not necessarily mean that you are wrong. There are many different approaches to the treatment of patients, and each case must be individualized based on the particular patient's circumstances. Appendixes C through G provide tables of average charges for hospital care, diagnostic imaging, clinical pathology diagnostic tests, miscellaneous services, and physician fees.

## Case 1

You are seeing Ted, a 52-year-old professor, with your preceptor. The patient has been diagnosed with mild (stage 1) hypertension, having blood pressure readings averaging 134/96 mm Hg on three different occasions. You decide to obtain some baseline data on the patient. Check the tests you would choose from the following list. Estimate their cost.

| Test | Cost |
|------|------|
| _____ Electrocardiogram (EKG) | _____ |
| _____ Chest x-ray (CXR) | _____ |
| _____ Exercise tolerance test (ETT) | _____ |
| _____ Holter monitor | _____ |
| _____ Urinalysis | _____ |
| _____ CBC count | _____ |
| _____ Chemistry screen | _____ |
| _____ Renal artery angiogram | _____ |
| **Total** | _____ |

After your workup is complete, you elect to begin antihypertensive drug therapy. Your preceptor asks you to write a prescription for a diuretic: hydrochlorothiazide (HCTZ), 25 mg/day. Having just reviewed *Cecil's Medicine Text*, you note that they recommend an angiotensin-converting enzyme (ACE) inhibitor for a white male in his 50s, and so suggest such treatment. Slightly embarrassed by this information, your preceptor quickly suggests placing the patient on captopril (Capoten), an ACE inhibitor that a very competent drug representative had recommended the previous week.

Despite treatment with captopril, the patient remains hypertensive on a follow-up visit 1 month later. You ask the patient if he is taking the medication. He admits to taking it only episodically. As it was so expensive, he explains, he thought that it might be too powerful to use every day.

Estimate the cost for a 1-month supply of captopril:_____

Estimate the cost for a 1-month supply of HCTZ:_____

Six months later, the patient returns complaining of chest pain and palpitations. You and your preceptor decide to perform a workup. You schedule the patient for the following tests. Check your choice(s), and estimate the cost for your workup.

| Test | Cost |
|---|---|
| _____ ETT | _____ |
| _____ Echocardiogram | _____ |
| _____ Thallium ETT | _____ |
| _____ Cardiac catheterization | _____ |
| _____ Holter monitor | _____ |
| **Total** | _____ |

You eventually diagnose a lesion of the left anterior descending (LAD) coronary artery, and the patient undergoes angioplasty. Estimate the cost for this procedure (hospital and physician charges): $_____.

Despite successful angioplasty, the patient leaves the hospital on several medications. Estimate his monthly expense for the following medications:

| Drug, dosage | Cost |
|---|---|
| Capoten (captopril), 25 mg tid | _____ |
| Cardizem (diltiazem), 60 mg qid | _____ |
| Persantine (dipyridamole), 75 mg tid | _____ |
| Pronestyl (procainamide), 375 mg tid | _____ |
| Nitroglycerin SL, 0.4 mg as needed | _____ |
| Prilosec (omeprazole), 20 mg qd | _____ |
| Glucotrol (glipizide), 10 mg qd | _____ |
| **Estimated total monthly drug cost:** | _____ |

With this cost in mind, estimate the monthly drug cost if you substitute some of the more expensive medications with less expensive alternatives:

| Drug, dosage | Cost |
| --- | --- |
| HCTZ, 25 mg qd, for Capoten | _____ |
| Nifedipine, 10 mg tid, for Cardizem | _____ |
| Cimetidine, 300 mg qd, for Prilosec | _____ |
| Tolbutamide, 250 mg qd, for Glucotrol | _____ |
| **Revised estimated monthly drug cost:** | _____ |
| **Total monthly savings:** | _____ |

Despite your aggressive treatment, the patient progressively worsens and 1 year later is admitted for coronary artery bypass graft (CABG) surgery. Estimate the hospital and surgical team charges: $_____.

A few weeks after discharge while opening his mail, the patient finds a bill for his CABG surgery, collapses, and is rushed to the emergency department by ambulance. Estimate the ambulance cost, including advanced life support (ALS) service with paramedics via a private company: $_____. Unfortunately, the patient dies in the emergency room from a severe myocardial infarction. Estimate the charges for the emergency room: $_____.

Though the patient has died, he continues to generate expenses associated with his condition. Estimate the cost of the funeral arrangements:

| | |
| --- | --- |
| Funeral | _____ |
| Cemetery plot and burial | _____ |
| Headstone | _____ |

On speaking to his wife, you learn that after his surgery, the patient had returned to his previous lifestyle and diet, proclaiming himself "good as new." What kind of programs could you have recommended to the patient to prevent him from relapsing into his unhealthy lifestyle? Estimate the cost of these programs.

## Case 2

You have just finished examining 30-month-old Jocelyn, who has a fever of 101.8°F and irritability, but who is otherwise okay. You determine that she has otitis media of the left ear. What organisms are the most likely to cause this infection?

What antibiotic therapy will you prescribe? Write the liquid form of this antibiotic.

---

**MED STUDENT ASSOCIATES**
**Not for Real Drugs**

NAME: _____ AGE: _____

ADDRESS: _____ DATE: _____

RX:

DEA# _____        _____ M.D.

PHYSICIAN'S SIGNATURE
Interchange is mandated unless the practitioner
writes the words "no substitution" in this space.

Repeat _____ Times
_____ Month

---

Estimate the cost of your treatment: $_____

You see the child at a follow-up examination 6 weeks later. At that time, her acute otitis media is resolved, but visible fluid remains behind her left tympanic membrane. Concerned about chronic serous otitis, you decide to treat prophylactically. What therapy do you recommend? Estimate the cost.

The mother is concerned about her daughter's hearing, and you request a formal hearing test (Behavioral Audiometry). Estimate the cost: $_____.

The fluid remains, and you consult an otolaryngologist for the placement of typanostomy tubes. Estimate the cost of this procedure, including the surgeon's fee: $_____.

## Case 3

You examine Greg, a 27-year-old male medical student who has hurt his back while doing landscaping for his summer job. Responding to the taunts of "bookworm" by his co-workers, he attempted to lift a heavy 20-lb bag of fertilizer, causing injury. He complains of recurrent lower back pain and has been to see a chiropractor, but his pain persists. You request x-rays of the lumbosacral region of the spine. Estimate the cost: $_____.

The x-rays are negative, and you decide to prescribe some medication to relieve his discomfort. Having just completed a rotation in the sports medicine clinic, Greg requests Orudis (ketoprofen). A drug representative had sponsored a luncheon and noted that Orudis was the drug of choice for musculoskeletal injuries. He claimed that because of its green packaging, Orudis had been adopted by the Celtics basketball team as their favorite pain medication, and that Larry Bird used it exclusively for his low back pain.

You give Greg a prescription for a 10-day supply. Pleased, he heads to the pharmacy. Estimate the cost for this prescription: $_____.

A short while later, you receive a call from Greg; it seems he cannot afford the medication. Chagrined, he requests a less expensive alternative. Write your choice of pain medication on page 102, and estimate its cost.

Estimate the cost: $_____.

Greg returns in one week, unimproved and convinced that he has a disk problem because he has developed some sciatica. He asks you to order a magnetic resonance imag-

```
┌─────────────────────────────────────────────────────┐
│              MED STUDENT ASSOCIATES                  │
│                Not for Real Drugs                    │
│                                                       │
│  NAME: _____      AGE: _____      │
│  ADDRESS: _____      DATE: _____      │
│  RX:                                                  │
│                                                       │
│  DEA# _____          _____ M.D.       │
│                           PHYSICIAN'S SIGNATURE       │
│                           Interchange is mandated unless the practitioner │
│                           writes the words "no substitution" in this space. │
│                                                       │
│  Repeat _____ Times                                   │
│         _____ Month                                   │
│                                                       │
└─────────────────────────────────────────────────────┘
```

ing (MRI) examination. Estimate the cost of the MRI: $_____. The MRI reveals no disk damage or abnormalities. What will you do now?

## Case 4

You are examining 10-year-old Danny in the emergency room. He was trying to catch turtles and fell into a dirty pond, twisting his ankle and cutting his foot on a piece of glass. The nursing staff has had the foot soaking in povidone-iodine (Betadine) solution. You irrigate the wound with normal saline and close with sutures. The mother is concerned about infection because the pond water is extremely muddy. What organisms are you most concerned about?

What prophylactic regimen will you prescribe?

Once the wound has been cleaned and treated, you request an x-ray of the twisted ankle. Estimate the cost: $_____. The x-ray is negative, and you write a prescription for a pain medication. Write your choice of pain medication below, and estimate its cost.

---

**MED STUDENT ASSOCIATES**
**Not for Real Drugs**

NAME: _____ AGE: _____

ADDRESS: _____ DATE: _____

RX:

DEA# _____ _____ M.D.

PHYSICIAN'S SIGNATURE
Interchange is mandated unless the practitioner
writes the words "no substitution" in this space.

Repeat _____ Times
_____ Month

---

Estimate the cost: $_____.

Estimate the total cost for this minor accident, which undoubtedly would have been prevented had Danny listened to his mother's request that he not play near the pond.

## Case 5

Jim, a 40-year-old teacher, comes in complaining of fatigue, nausea, occasional vomiting, and loose stools for 2 weeks. He complains of feelings of abdominal fullness and occasional pain over his epigastrium and right upper quadrant (RUQ). On physical examination, you find Jim to be in relatively good health except for a low-grade temperature, mild obesity, and some RUQ tenderness, and his liver percusses to a span of 12 cm.

What are you considering for his diagnosis? What diagnostic testing will you obtain? Estimate the cost for each diagnostic test that you will obtain as part of your initial workup.

The laboratory studies reveal elevated liver function tests (LFTs). How will you follow up? Estimate the cost for your workup.

The final results are consistent with cholelithiasis. Gallstones are detected, but the patient does not want surgery, as he is worried about having an ugly scar and he has no sick days at his work. He will have to use his vacation time to have the operation. You recommend laparoscopic surgery, as it leaves a much smaller scar, costs less (estimate cost: $_____), and he will only miss a few days of work compared to the several weeks usually lost after undergoing a traditional cholecystectomy. Estimate the cost, including the surgeon's fee: $_____.

## Case 6

Anthony, an 8-year-old patient, comes into your office complaining of shortness of breath and wheezing. After your thorough examination, the findings of which are essentially normal other than scattered rhonchi and diffuse wheezing, you decide to order some diagnostic tests. Choose the tests you would order from the list below; estimate the cost.

| Test | Cost |
| --- | --- |
| _____ Pulmonary function test | _____ |
| _____ Chest x-ray | _____ |
| _____ CBC count | _____ |
| _____ Allergy testing | _____ |
| _____ Blood gas | _____ |
| _____ Oxygen saturation | _____ |

What is your diagnosis? What will you prescribe? Estimate the cost for your therapy.

If you decide to prescribe an inhaler, write the prescription below:

---

**MED STUDENT ASSOCIATES**
**Not for Real Drugs**

NAME: _____  AGE: _____

ADDRESS: _____  DATE: _____

RX:

DEA#_____     _____ M.D.

PHYSICIAN'S SIGNATURE
Interchange is mandated unless the practitioner
writes the words "no substitution" in this space.

Repeat _____ Times
_____ Month

---

The patient returns with continued wheezing. His mother requests allergy-testing as she is concerned that their new cat may be causing the problem, so you refer him for allergy-testing. Estimate the cost for a standard skin-patch test for environmental allergens: $_____.

The patient tests positive for feline allergy, and you place him on immunotherapy—monthly injections of cat allergen to diminish his allergic response. Estimate the annual cost for his allergy immunotherapy: $_____.

## Case 7

You are seeing Kate, a 26-year-old previously healthy student who has had symptoms of dysuria and frequency for 2 days. She denies other problems and her last menstrual period was 1 week ago. On examination, she is afebrile, without flank tenderness, and otherwise appears well. What workup will you obtain? Estimate the cost.

What diagnosis are you considering? What therapy will you prescribe? Estimate the cost.

The patient returns monthly with recurrent urinary tract infections. Given this chronic course, what further workup will you order, and what further treatment will you suggest? Again, estimate the cost.

## Case 8

Mary, a 39-year-old secretary, presents with complaints of severe headaches. She has been a patient of yours for a long time and you have seen her for routine care and episodic problems. She complained of a similar headache 3 years previously, but it had resolved and this is essentially a new complaint for her. She notes that the headaches are pounding in nature, and seem to settle around her eyes, although frequently it seems as though she has a tight band around her head. She points to a spot on the back of her skull where the pain seems particularly severe. The headaches have occurred almost daily over the last couple of weeks. On further questioning, she reports that she does not awaken with the headaches; they seem to come on gradually during the day and are particularly severe by the end of the workday. She goes home and takes some aspirin, which provides minimal relief. Mary is able to get to sleep without difficulty and sleeps through the night. Indeed, she relates that rather than the headaches keeping her up, she feels exhausted at the end of the day and has no problem falling asleep. Her review of systems is otherwise negative. She denies any visual changes, numbness, or weakness. The results of a physical examination are essentially within normal limits, with cranial nerves being intact and a funduscopic examination demonstrating normal findings. What diagnostic and/or therapeutic modalities will you employ at this point? Estimate the costs.

The patient returns for follow-up in 2 weeks. She reports that the medication you prescribed has helped in relieving the headaches; however, she is concerned that she continues to have them daily. At this point, she expresses her worries about the possibility of a brain tumor and requests that some x-rays be taken or a brain scan performed to be sure that this is not the case. Estimate the cost of a computed tomography (CT) scan of the head: $_____; or MRI scan of the brain: $_____. What will you do now?

## Case 9

You are taking care of Peter, a 33-year-old horticultural executive who comes in to see you complaining of what he describes as heartburn. On further questioning, you learn that he has a sharp burning sensation in his epigastrium and substernally. Occasionally, he has a sour taste in the back of his mouth. His symptoms are so severe that they occasionally wake him up from sleep, for which he gets up and has a glass of warm milk and the symptoms seem to resolve. He notes there has been increasing pressure at work, and he has been exploring starting his own business. He otherwise feels well and other than having been seen in the past for routine health visits, his past medical history is benign. He denies problems with vomiting, or diarrhea, or melena. He keeps fit as he has a physically demanding job. He does admit to drinking several cans of Coke on a daily basis and occasionally has a beer or two prior to retiring in the evening. His alcohol intake has increased as of late, as he has begun a new hobby of making his own home brew.

His vital signs are normal. The results of a physical examination are within normal limits, but there is some mild tenderness to palpation over the epigastrium. Given the history and results of physical examination, you feel quite comfortable that his symptoms are not cardiac in nature but limited to the gastrointestinal tract. What diagnostic and therapeutic measures will you undertake at this time? Estimate the cost.

# REFERENCES

AMA Council on Ethical and Judicial Affairs. Ethical issues in managed care. JAMA 1995;273:330–335.

Azevedo, D. Oregon update: If this is rationing, what's the problem? Med Econ 1995;17:144–159.

Balinsky, W. The Impact of DRGs of the Healthcare Industry. Health Care Rev 1987;12: 61–74.

Barry HC, Ebell MH, Hickhner J. Evaluation of suspected urinary tract infection in ambulatory women: A cost-utility analysis of office-based strategies. J Fam Pract 1997;44:48–53.

Baumgart AJ. Quality through health policy: The Canadian example. International Nurs Rev 1993;40:167–170.

Bell CW. Managed care: Update and future directions. J Ambul Manage 1990;13: 15–26.

Berger JT, Rosner F. The ethics of practice guidelines. Arch Intern Med 1996;156: 2051–2056.

Bodenheimer T. The HMO backlash—righteous or reactionary? Sounding Board 1996;335:1601–1603.

Bowling A. Management. Setting priorities in health: The Oregon experiment. Nurs Stand 1992;6:28–30.

Bristow LR. The corporatization of healthcare. Colo Med 1993;90:358–361.

Butcher RO. Managed care now and forever. J Natl Med Assoc 1993;85(7):505–507.

Caroll MS. Managed care programs: An employer perspective. Top Health Care Financ 1993;20:10–16.

Clancy CM, Brody H. Managed care, Jekyll or Hyde? JAMA 1995;273:338–339.

Crawshaw R. The Oregon Medicaid controversy. N Engl J Med 1992;327:642–644.

Curtiss FR. Managed care: The second generation. Am J Hosp Pharm 1990;47:2047–2052.

Ellwood PM, Lundberg GD. Managed care: A work in progress. JAMA 1996;276:1083–1086.

Fabian T, Kincses G. Review of the financing system of prospective payments/diagnosis related groups, based on experience in the USA. Orv Hetil 1993;134:523–526.

Family Practice Management (ISSN 1069–5648). Published by The American Academy of Family Physicians, 8880 Ward Parkway, Kansas City, MO 64114-2797. (phone 1-800-274-2237).

Gilbert FI Jr. The case for restructuring healthcare in the U.S.: The Hawaii Paradigm. J Med Syst 1993;17:283–288.

Gore A Jr. National policy prospective:Oregon's bold mistake. Acad Med 1990;65:634–635.

Grumbach K, Bodenheimer T. Health care policy: A clinical approach—mechanisms for controlling costs. JAMA 1995;273:1223–1230.

Hayes GJ. Physicians who have practiced in both the United States and Canada compare the systems. Am J Public Health 1993;83:1544–1548.

Hillman AL. Contractual arrangements between HMO's and primary care physicians. Med Care 1992;30:36–47.

Honigsbaum F. The evolution of the (British) NHS. BMG 1990;301:694–699.

Hoy EW. Changes and growth in managed care. Health Aff 1991;10:18–36.

Hsiao WC, et al. An overview of the development and refinement of the resource based relative value scale. The Foundation for Reform of U.S. Physician Payment. Med Care 1992;30(11 suppl):NS 1–12, NS 61–79.

Hsiao WC. Comparing healthcare systems: What nations can learn from one another. J Health Polit Policy Law 1992;17:613–616.

Hunter DJ. Doctors as managers: Poachers turned gamekeepers. Soc Sci Med 1992;35:557–566.

Iglehart JK. The American healthcare system—introduction. N Engl J Med 1992;326:962–967.

Iglehart JK. The American healthcare system—managed care. N Engl J Med 1992;327:742–747.

Iglehart JK. The American healthcare system—Medicare. N Engl J Med 1992;327:1467–1472.

Iglehart JK. The American healthcare system—private insurance. N Engl J Med 1992;320:1715–1720.

Iglehart JK. Health systems in three nations. Health Aff 1991;10:254–261. 1991 Fall.

Jacobs MO. Physician characteristics and training emphasis—Considered desirable by leaders of HMO's. J Med Ed 1987;62:725–731.

Jensen HL. The impact of managed care on physicians. Qual Assur Util Rev 1991;6:109–114.

Johnson J. Managed care in the 1990's: Providers' new role for innovative health delivery. Hospitals 1992;66:26–30.

Kronick R. The marketplace in healthcare reform—The demographic limitations of managed competition. N Engl J Med 1993;328:148–152.

Letsch S. National healthcare spending in 1991. Health Aff 1993;12:94–104.

Levin JC. Reflections on national healthcare reform based on Hawaii's experience. Am J Surg 1994;167:227–231.

Levy JM. Understanding the Medicare fee schedule and its impact on physicians under the final rule. Med Care 1992;30(11 suppl):NS 80–94.

Loewy EH. Guidelines, managed care, and ethics. Arch Intern Med 1996;156:2038–2040.

Maxwell JG. Changes in Britain's health care: An American attempts to revisit from the London post. JAMA 1996;275:789–793.

Medical Economics. Published by The Medical Economics Company, 5 Paragon Drive, Montvale, NJ 07645–1742. (phone 1-800-232-7379).

The Medical Letter (ISSN 0025-732X). 100 Main Street, New Rochelle, NY 10801-7537. (phone 1-800-211-2769).

Montague J. MD's in the middle: Managed care and looming reform put the squeeze on many middle-aged physicians. Hosp Health Net 1994;68:52, 54.

Newbauer D. State model: A pioneer in health system reform. Health Aff 1993;12:31–39.

Osterweis M, McLaughlin CJ, Manasse HR, Hopper CL, eds. Washington, DC: The U.S. Health Workforce, Power, Politics, and Policy. AHC, 1996.

Shameso B. The United States should be wary of Canada's healthcare system. Can Med Assoc J 1992;146:2046–2048.

Simborg D. DRG Creep. N Engl J Med 1981;304:1602–1604.

Steinbrook R. The Oregon Medicaid demonstration project—will it provide adequate medical care? N Engl J Med 1992;325:340–343.

Vogel DE. Family physicians and managed care, A View to the 90's. Kansas City:Am Acad Fam Phys, 1992.

Weiner JP. Primary care delivery in the U.S. and four northwest European countries. Milbank Q 1987;65:426–459.

Woolhandler S, Himmelstein D. Extreme risk—The new corporate proposition for physicians. N Engl J Med 1995;333:1706–1708.

# GLOSSARY

## Alliance

A nonprofit or state agency that provides consumers in its areas with information about health insurance plans and negotiates with insurers to obtain better rates.

## Balance Billing

The practice of a provider billing a patient for all charges not paid for by the insurance plan. Some states and most managed care plans prohibit providers from balance billing, except for copayments and deductibles.

## Capitated Plan

Managed care plan pays a physician a fixed amount to care for a patient over a given time period. For example, a primary care physician is paid a fixed amount every month for each patient enrolled in the plan, regardless of whether he or she sees the patient. However, providers do not receive additional payments, even if the costs of care exceed the fixed amount.

## Cost Containment

The process by which control over the rising costs of health care are kept in check.

## Cost Effective

A term that refers to the allocation of resources in a manner intended to maximize outcome and minimize cost.

## Deductible

The initial amount that the consumer must first pay for medical services before the third-party payer pays the remaining amount in a given period of time.

## Diagnosis-Related Groups (DRGs)

A statistical system of classifying an inpatient stay into groups for purposes of payment under the Medicare system.

## Disease Management

Provision of complete patient care, typically by specialists, for certain diseases, such as cancer therapy or transplantation care.

## Employer Mandate

A requirement that employers offer and pay for their employee's insurance.

## Fee For Service (FFS)

An established fee paid for each service provided by the physician. This is the traditional way physicians have been paid. The more services provided, the more the physician is paid.

## Gatekeeper

A nonmedical, though widely used term that refers to a primary care case-management type of health plan.

## Group Practice

The American Medical Association defines group practice as three or more physicians who deliver patient care, make joint use of equipment and personnel, and divide income by a pre-arranged formula.

## Health Maintenance Organization (HMO)

HMOs are organized health-care systems that are responsible for both the financing and delivery of a broad range of comprehensive health services to an enrolled population for a prepaid fixed fee.

## Independent Practice Association (IPA)

An IPA, known also as an individual practice association, is an association of individual, independent physicians or a small group or physicians that has been formed for the purpose of contracting with one or more managed health-care organizations.

## Integrated Delivery System (IDS)

Strategic alliances between physicians and hospitals that assure shared risk through common ownership, governance, shared revenues, capital, planning, and management. The goal of an IDS is to provide a planned, coordinated, collaborative process that maximizes the efficient allocation of resources providing high-quality health care.

## Length of Stay (LOS)

Duration of a patient's hospital stay, expressed in days.

## Managed Competition

The concept that economic incentives are primary determinants of how consumers and providers use health care and that by changing market incentives, reform will follow.

## Managed Health Care

Managed care is the coordinated delivery of cost-effective health-care services. Managed care organizations call this "The right care, in the right place, at the right time."

## Mandate

Requirements established by state or federal standards. For example, all employers with more than 25 employees that offer health insurance must also offer an HMO plan as an alternative.

## Medicaid

A program administered by the state government to provide health insurance for people who live in poverty. Funding is provided by both the federal and state government. There are no premiums.

## Medical Malpractice Liability Insurance

1. Occurrence Coverage: Covers the physician for cases occurring during the coverage period. If the patient sues after the physician has canceled the insurance policy, but the patient's suit refers to the time that the physician was covered by the policy, then the occurrence policy will cover the physician.
2. Claim-Made Coverage: Less expensive than occurrence coverage, but only covers the physician for claims made during the time that the policy is in effect. Wise physicians avoid this type of insurance or purchase a policy to cover claims after the claim-made coverage has expired, though this tail policy is expensive.

### Medicare

A program administered and funded by the federal government to provide health insurance for people 65 years and older and some younger disabled people. Medicare has two parts: Part A pays for hospital care, and Part B pays for physician care. Medicare hospital insurance (Part A) does not charge a premium if you have sufficient work credits under Social Security. Medicare medical insurance (Part B) charges a premium. Medicare does not cover everything. For example, the medical insurance only pays for 80% of the allowed physician fee. The patient is responsible for a copayment equal to 20% of the allowed fee. There are also deductibles and restrictions for hospital care.

### National Health Service (NHS)

Socialized medical program of Great Britain.

### Open Access Plans

Managed care plans that do not require patients to have an assigned primary care physician acting as a gatekeeper; rather, patients can self refer to specialists.

### Open-Enrollment Period

The period when an employee may change health plans, usually occurs once a year.

### Peer Review Organization (PRO)

A panel of physicians who review the diagnoses of cases for quality and appropriateness of care. PROs typically contract to review cases for Medicare.

### Physician-Organized Delivery Systems (PODS)

Small groups of physicians who contract together with managed care organizations in risk-sharing agreements to provide total care for a capitated pool of patients.

### Point of Service

A plan wherein members do not have to choose how to receive services until they need them. The most common use of the term applies to plans that permit members to go outside the plan for services, with additional charges to be paid by subscribers.

## Preferred-Provider Arrangement (PPA)

A PPA is usually the same as a PPO. However, some use the term PPA to describe a less formal relationship than would be described by a PPO. PPO infers that an organization exists, whereas a PPA may be an informal arrangement among providers and payers.

## Preferred-Provider Organization (PPO)

A group of physicians that, together with a hospital, provide services to a patient pool. These health-care providers, selected by managed-care organizations or insurance companies, act as a PPO while maintaining their individuality. The managed care organizations or insurance companies obtain a fee discount from the providers in exchange for a guaranteed pool of patients.

## Primary Care Physician

A physician who practices general internal medicine, family medicine, or general pediatrics.

## Resource-Based Relative Value System (RBRVS)

System used by Medicare to reimburse physicians.

## Risk-Sharing Plan

Contractual arrangement in which physicians share financial risk with the managed care organization for the cost of the medical care delivered to their panel of patients. Under such plans, if the cost of care exceeds the budget, the physician has to help cover this loss.

## Single-Payer System

Instead of paying insurance premiums for health care, individuals pay some type of tax to support a national health-care system (e.g., Canadian-style health-care system).

## Solo Practice

A private practice run by a single physician.

## Specialist

Someone who is recognized to have expertise in a specialty of medicine or surgery. Within health maintenance organizations, it usually refers to physicians who receive referrals from primary care physicians.

## Standard Benefits Package

A defined set of services and goods, such as inpatient care, preventive treatment, and drugs, that all insurance plans must offer.

## Traditional Indemnity Plan

Health-care insurance that reimburses the patient for fees they have paid. Blue Cross/Blue Shield is an example of this type of plan. Payment is predominantly for procedural services.

## Utilization Review

A review of the appropriateness of a service before, during, and after a hospitalization or outpatient surgery.

## Withhold

A portion of a physician's payment that is set aside to the end of the contract year. At that time, use of services are examined. If use is higher than expected, some or all of the withhold is not given to the physician. Withholding payments to the end of the contract year is one form of risk-sharing.

# APPENDIXES

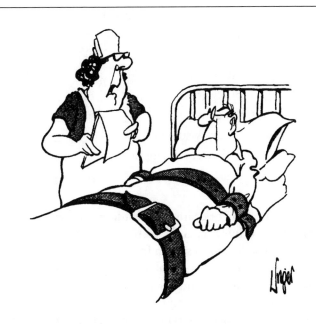

*"Hospital regulations. You gotta wear the straps while I read the bill."*

# A. ANSWERS TO PROBLEM-SOLVING CASES

## Case 1

You are seeing Ted, a 52-year-old professor, with your preceptor. The patient has been diagnosed with mild (stage 1) hypertension, having blood pressure readings averaging 134/96 mm Hg on three different occasions. You decide to obtain some baseline data on the patient. Check the tests you would choose from the following list. Estimate their cost.

| | Test | Cost |
|---|---|---|
| __X__ | Electrocardiogram (EKG) | $ 86 |
| _____ | Chest x-ray (CXR) | 169 |
| _____ | Exercise tolerance test (ETT) | 532 |
| _____ | Holter monitor | 150 |
| __X__ | Urinalysis | 27 |
| __X__ | CBC count | 23 |
| __X__ | Chemistry screen | 200 |
| _____ | Renal artery angiogram | $1590 |
| | Total | $ 336 |

Baseline labwork should include a CBC count, chemistry screen, urinalysis, and an EKG for a total cost of $336. These tests will help to screen for other risk factors of coronary artery disease (e.g., diabetes, hyperlipidemia) and to look for evidence of end-organ damage (e.g., proteinuria, left ventricular hypertrophy). The other tests are not routinely recommended. A renal artery angiogram would rule out renal artery stenosis as a cause of hypertension, but this is rare (0.5%) and the patient would present differently (higher readings, difficulty achieving control, etc.).

After your workup is complete, you elect to begin anti-hypertensive drug therapy. Your preceptor asks you to write a prescription for a diuretic: hydrochlorothiazide (HCTZ), 25 mg/day. Having just reviewed *Cecil's Medicine Text*, you note that they recommend an angiotensin-converting enzyme (ACE) inhibitor for a white male in his 50s, and so suggest such treatment. Slightly embarrassed by this information, your preceptor quickly suggests placing the patient on captopril (Capoten), an ACE inhibitor that a very competent drug representative had recommended the previous week.

Despite treatment with captopril, the patient remains hypertensive on a follow-up visit 1 month later. You ask the patient if he is taking the medication. He admits to taking it only episodically. As it was so expensive, he explains, he thought that it might be too powerful to use every day.

Estimate the cost for a 1-month supply of captopril: <u>$52.00</u>

Estimate the cost for a 1-month supply of HCTZ: <u>$ 3.50</u>

**There has been an increase in the use of ACE inhibitors and calcium channel blocking agents for the treatment of hypertension over the last few years. However, there is no substantive evidence to justify large-scale avoidance of diuretics and beta-blockers in the treatment of hypertension. Although side effects occur in a small percentage of patients, they can be watched for and may be avoided by decreasing dosages used. Indeed, the latest report of the Joint National Committee on High Blood Pressure (1993) continues to recommend diuretics or beta-blockers as first-step choices.**

Six months later, the patient returns complaining of chest pain and palpitations. You and your preceptor decide to perform a workup. You schedule the patient for the following tests. Check your choice(s), and estimate the cost for your workup.

| | Test | Cost |
|---|---|---|
| __X__ | ETT | $ 532 |
| _____ | Echocardiogram | 500 |
| _____ | Thallium ETT | 1660 |
| _____ | Cardiac catheterization | 3752 |
| _____ | Holter monitor | 150 |
| | Total | $ 532 |

An ETT ($532) would be appropriate at this time and, given the history, would most likely be positive indicating coronary artery disease. Additionally, a Holter monitor might be ordered because of the complaints of palpitations, although any dysrhythmia might show up with the ETT. A cardiac catheterization to view the coronary arteries would be appropriate as a preoperative step, that is, if the patient failed medical therapy and was being considered for angioplasty or coronary artery bypass graft (CABG) surgery.

You eventually diagnose a lesion of the left anterior descending (LAD) coronary artery, and the patient undergoes angioplasty. Estimate cost for this procedure (hospital and physician charges): **$12,750**.

Despite successful angioplasty, the patient leaves the hospital on several medications. Estimate his monthly expense for the following medications:

| Drug, dosage | Cost |
|---|---|
| Capoten (captopril), 25 mg tid | $ 52 |
| Cardizem (diltiazem), 60 mg qid | 74 |
| Persantine (dipyridamole), 75 mg tid | 56 |
| Pronestyl (procainamide), 375 mg tid | 13 |
| Nitroglycerin SL, 0.4 mg as needed | 6 |
| Prilosec (omeprazole), 20 mg qd | 97 |
| Glucotrol (glipizide), 10 mg qd | 21 |
| **Estimated total monthly drug cost:** | **$ 319** |

With this cost in mind, estimate the monthly drug cost if you substitute some of the more expensive medications with less expensive alternatives:

| Drug, dosage | Cost |
|---|---|
| HCTZ, 25 mg qd, for Capoten | $ 3.50 |
| Nifedipine, 10 mg tid, for Cardizem | 25.00 |
| Cimetidine, 300 mg qd, for Prilosec | 19.00 |
| Tolbutamide, 250 mg qd, for Glucotrol | 6.00 |
| **Revised estimated monthly drug cost:** | $ 53.50 |
| **Total monthly savings:** | $266.50 |

Despite your aggressive treatment, the patient progressively worsens and 1 year later is admitted for CABG surgery. Estimate the hospital and surgical team charges: **$33,000.**

**The following is a summary example of hospital and physician's charges for an uncomplicated CABG surgery with 7 to 9 days of hospitalization:**

| | |
|---|---|
| **Cardiology** | $ 1056 |
| **Nursing, operating room** | 1025 |
| **Nursing, recovery room** | 450 |
| **Pulmonary laboratoryoratory** | 1574 |
| **Respiratory care** | 1250 |
| **Pharmacy** | 2385 |
| **Radiology** | 985 |
| **Anesthesia supplies** | 2705 |
| **General supplies** | 1900 |
| **Clinical pathology blood bank** (units of blood) | 1200 |
| **Clinical pathology** (ABGs during surgery) | 3200 |
| **Room charge (semiprivate $575/day)** | 3450 |
| **Room charge, ICU ($1400/day)** | 4200 |
| **Surgeon's fee** | 6500 |
| **Anesthesiologist's fee (215 minutes)** | 1900 |
| **Total:** | $33,780 |

A few weeks after discharge while opening his mail, the patient finds a bill for his CABG surgery, collapses, and is rushed to the emergency department by ambulance. Estimate the ambulance cost, including advanced life support (ALS) service with paramedics via a private company: **$450**. Unfortunately, the patient dies in the emergency room from a severe myocardial infarction. Estimate the charges for the emergency room: **$1350**.

Though the patient has died, he continues to generate expenses associated with his fatal condition. Estimate the cost of the funeral arrangements:

| | |
|---|---|
| Funeral | **$4000** |
| Cemetery plot and burial | **$ 650** |
| Headstone | **$1000** |

On speaking to his wife, you learn that after his surgery, the patient had returned to his previous lifestyle and diet, proclaiming himself "good as new" (Figure A.1). What kind of programs could you have recommended to the patient to prevent him from relapsing into this unhealthy lifestyle? Estimate the cost of these programs.

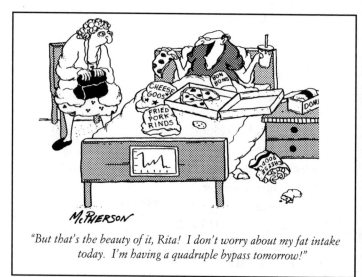

"But that's the beauty of it, Rita! I don't worry about my fat intake today. I'm having a quadruple bypass tomorrow!"

**Figure A.1**

Lifestyle modification includes weight reduction; changing diets to decrease sodium, fats, and cholesterol; modifying alcohol intake; increasing physical activity; and avoiding smoking. These measures are extremely important and should be tended to as initial therapy and reiterated continually. A nutritionist and tobacco cessation groups should be utilized. These typically cost less than $100.

## Case 2

You have just finished examining 30-month-old Jocelyn, who has a fever of 101.8°F and irritability, but who is otherwise okay. You determine that she has otitis media of the left ear. What organisms are the most likely to cause this infection?

Otitis media in a child is most likely caused by the following organisms:

| | |
|---|---|
| 30 – 50% | *Streptococcus pneumoniae* |
| 20 – 30% | **Virus** |
| 20 – 30% | *Haemophilus influenzae* |
| 5 – 15% | *Branhamella catarrhalis* |
| 2 – 5% | **Beta-hemolytic streptococci, group A** |
| 2 – 5% | *Staphylococcus aureus* |

What antibiotic therapy will you prescribe? Write the liquid form of this antibiotic.

---

**MED STUDENT ASSOCIATES**
Not for Real Drugs

NAME:  Jocelyn                          AGE:    2¹ᐟ²

ADDRESS:                                DATE:

RX: Amoxicillin 205 mg/5 ml #150 cc
     Sig: 1 tsp tid

DEA# _____                      _____ M.D.

PHYSICIAN'S SIGNATURE
Interchange is mandated unless the practitioner
writes the words "no substitution" in this space.

Repeat ___0___ Times
          _____ Month

---

Estimate the cost of your treatment:  **$8.62**.

**Amoxicillin is an appropriate first-line treatment and sulfamethoxazole-trimethoprim (Bactrim) can be prescribed for the penicillin-allergic patient. Approximately 30% of *H. influenzae* and *B. catarrhalis* organisms produce beta-lactamase. Therefore, some recommend prescribing a beta-lactamase–resistant antibiotic for the initial choice. Given the cost differential, it makes sense to use the less expensive amoxicillin first, reserving the expensive beta-lactamase–resistant antibiotics for the small percentage of children who do not respond because of a presumed beta-lactamase–producing micro-organism. Table A.1 lists the commonly prescribed antibiotics for otitis media and their cost.**

You see the child at a follow-up examination 6 weeks later. At that time, her acute otitis media is resolved, but visible fluid remains behind her left tympanic membrane. Concerned about chronic serous otitis, you decide to treat prophylactically. What therapy do you recommend? Estimate the cost.

**A 3-month supply of Gantrisin (sulfisoxazole), 500 mg qd costs $13.**

The mother is concerned about her daughter's hearing, and you request a formal hearing test (Behavioral Audi-

## SOME ANTIMICROBIALS FOR ACUTE OTITIS MEDIA

| Drug | Daily Dosage | Cost[a] |
|------|-------------|------|
| Amoxicillin – average generic price (*Amoxil*–SK Beecham) | 40 mg/kg in 3 doses | $ 6.02<br><br>6.10 |
| Amoxicillin-clavulanic acid<br><br>(*Augmentin*–SK Beecham) | 40 mg/kg amoxicillin 10 mg/kg clavulanic acid in 3 doses | 48.10 |
| Cefaclor (*Ceclor*–Lilly) | 40 mg/kg in 2 or 3 doses | 51.78 |
| Cefixime (*Suprax*–Lederle) | 8 mg/kg in 1 or 2 doses | 45.66 |
| Cefprozil (*Cefzil*–Bristol) | 30 mg/kg in 2 doses | 45.59 |
| Cefuroxime axetil (*Ceftin*[b]–Allen/Hanburys) | 500 mg in 2 doses | 62.84 |
| Cefpodoxime (*Vantin* – Upjohn) | 10 mg/kg in 2 doses | 54.00 |
| Erythromycin-sulfisoxazole – average generic price (*Pediazole*–Ross/Abbott) | 50 mg/kg erythromycin– 150 mg/kg sulfisoxazole in 4 doses | 22.77<br><br>30.08 |
| Loracarbef (*Lorabid*–Lilly) | 30 mg/kg in 2 doses | 56.40 |
| Trimethoprim-sulfamethoxazole – average generic price (*Bactrim*–Roches) (*Septra*–Burroughs Wellcome) | 8 mg/kg TMP–40 mg/kg SMX in 2 doses | 3.43<br><br>12.83<br>12.26 |

■ **Table A.1**

[a] *Cost to the pharmacist as packaged for 10 days' treatment of a 15-kg child, according to Average Wholesale Price listings in* Red Book *1993 and February 1994* Update.
[b] *Currently available only in tablets in the United States.*
*Source: Drugs for treatment of acute otitis media in children.* Med Lett Drugs Ther *1994;36:19–20.*

ometry). Estimate the cost: **$50**.

The fluid remains, and you consult an otolaryngologist for the placement of tympanostomy tubes. Estimate the cost of this procedure, including the surgeon's fee: **$1150**.

## Case 3

You examine Greg, a 27-year-old male medical student who has hurt his back while doing landscaping for his summer job. Responding to the taunts of "bookworm" by his co-workers, he attempted to lift a heavy 20-lb bag of fertilizer, causing injury. He complains of recurrent lower back pain and has been to see a chiropractor, but his pain persists. You request x-rays of the lumbosacral region of the spine. Estimate the cost: **$162**.

The x-rays are negative, and you decide to prescribe some medication to relieve his discomfort. Having just completed a rotation in the sports medicine clinic, Greg requests Orudis (ketoprofen). A drug representative had sponsored a luncheon and noted that Orudis was the drug of choice for musculoskeletal injuries. Because of its green packaging, the representative had claimed that Orudis had been adopted by the Celtics basketball team as their favorite pain medication, and that Larry Bird used it exclusively for his low back pain.

You give Greg a prescription for a 10-day supply. Pleased, he heads to the pharmacy. Estimate the cost for this prescription: **$31**.

A short while later you receive a call from Greg; it seems he cannot afford the medication. Chagrined, he requests a less expensive alternative. Write your choice of pain medication below, and estimate its cost.

---

**MED STUDENT ASSOCIATES**
**Not for Real Drugs**

NAME: __Greg_____          AGE: ___27____

ADDRESS: _____          DATE: _____

RX: **Ibuprofen 600 mg #30**
     **Sig: 1 tid with food prn**

DEA# _____                        _____ M.D.

                                    PHYSICIAN'S SIGNATURE
                                    Interchange is mandated unless the practitioner
                                    writes the words "no substitution" in this space.

Repeat ___1___ Times
        _____ Month

Estimate the cost: **$3.40**.

**Nonsteroidal anti-inflammatory drugs (NSAIDS) are commonly prescribed for musculoskeletal injuries. The price range for these medications is considerable, from over-the-counter aspirin ($1.99/100 tablets) to Orudis (ketoprofen) ($31/30 tablets). Figure A.2 outlines the costs for these medications.**

**In addition to NSAIDs, a muscle relaxant is frequently prescribed if there is muscle spasm detected on examination. Some commonly prescribed muscle relaxants include:**

| | |
|---|---|
| **Diazepam (Valium)** | **$ 1.48/30 tablets** |
| **Flexeril** | **$21.86/30 tablets** |

Greg returns in 1 week, unimproved and convinced that he has a disk problem because he has developed some sciatica. He asks you to order a magnetic resonance imaging (MRI) examination. Estimate the cost of the

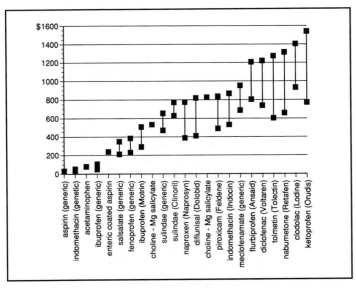

**Figure A.2** *Costs for nonsteroidal anti-inflammatory drugs. (Costs calculated in 1994, based on one year of use.)*

MRI: <u>**$1437**</u>. The MRI reveals no disk damage or abnormalities. What will you do now?

**Ninety percent of patients with low back pain will have resolution of their symptoms in 4 weeks, regardless of therapy. Therefore, assuming that the patient's history and physical findings are consistent with muscle strain of the lumbosacral region, there is no need to obtain any diagnostic imaging studies initially. Such studies should be reserved for the elderly patient, or for the patient whose problem does not resolve in 4 weeks or who has initial findings consistent with nerve root compression or more significant pathology.**

**When back pain continues, an appropriate referral would be for physical therapy to teach the patient stretching and strengthening exercises, and appropriate back hygiene. This will help to speed healing and prevent recurrences.**

## Case 4

You are examining 10-year-old Danny in the emergency department. He was trying to catch turtles and fell into the dirty pond, twisting his ankle and cutting his foot on a piece of glass. The nursing staff has had the foot soaking in povidone-iodine (Betadine) solution. You irrigate the wound with normal saline and close with sutures. The mother is concerned about infection because of the extremely muddy water in the pond. What organisms are you most concerned about?

**Wounds can be contaminated with *Clostridium tetani*, as this bacillus lives in the soil. Sutured wounds can also become infected from normal skin bacteria—staphylococci and streptococci.**

What prophylactic regimen will you prescribe?

**Appropriate wound prophylaxis includes careful attention to cleansing the wound and debridement of dead tissue prior to suturing. Irrigation with normal saline solution is sufficient for cleansing. Sutures should be removed**

as soon as possible (5–7 days), as they represent a foreign body that could become a site for infection. The patient's immunization status should be checked, and diphtheria-tetanus immunization administered, if needed. It is not necessary to prescribe an antibiotic if the above-mentioned treatment has been given. The patient should be instructed to watch for signs and symptoms of an infection and encouraged to return if there are concerns.

Once the wound has been cleaned and treated, you request an x-ray of the twisted ankle. Estimate the cost: **$100**. The x-ray is negative, and you write a prescription for a pain medication. Write your choice of pain medication below, and estimate its cost.

---

**MED STUDENT ASSOCIATES**
**Not for Real Drugs**

NAME:  Danny                AGE:      10

ADDRESS:                    DATE:

RX: **Ibuprofen 400 mg #30**
    **Sig: 1 tid with food prn**

DEA#                                              M.D.

PHYSICIAN'S SIGNATURE
Interchange is mandated unless the practitioner
writes the words "no substitution" in this space.

Repeat ___0___ Times
      _____ Month

---

Estimate the cost: **$4.20**.

Estimate the total cost for this minor accident, which undoubtedly would have been prevented had Anthony listened to his mother's request that he not play near the pond.

| | |
|---|---:|
| Emergency room charge | $110 |
| Emergency room physician | 100 |
| X-ray | 100 |
| Diphtheria-tetanus immunization | 8 |
| Broad-spectrum antibiotic (Keflex, cephalexin) | 14 |
| Pain medication (Naprosyn, naproxen) | 15 |
| Total | $347 |

An alternative scenario: Instead of coming into the emergency room, you tell the patient to come to your office. On careful examination, you feel the injury is consistent with a sprain and elect to treat it conservatively without taking x-rays. Because you know the patient, you do not prescribe any antibiotics but counsel to watch for signs and symptoms of infection and to call if they appear. You clean and suture the wound and prescribe ice packs and alternative pain medications such as Aspirin (cost: $1.99) or ibuprofen (cost: $3.99), both of which come as inexpensive over-the-counter generic versions. In addition, you do not give a diphtheria-tetanus shot because your office records reveal that his immunizations are up-to-date.

The cost for this office visit is $90 compared to the total cost for emergency room treatment plus aggressive pain and infection therapy of $346.

## Case 5

Jim, a 40-year-old teacher, comes in complaining of fatigue, nausea, occasional vomiting, and loose stools for 2 weeks. He complains of feelings of abdominal fullness and occasional pain over his epigastrium and right upper quadrant (RUQ). On physical examination, you find Jim to be in relatively good health except for a low-grade temperature, mild obesity, and some RUQ tenderness, and his liver percusses to a span of 12 cm.

What are you considering for his diagnosis? What diagnostic testing will you obtain? Estimate the cost for each diagnostic test that you will obtain as part of your initial workup.

**The presentation and examination suggest that the patient has either hepatitis or cholecystitis. Appropriate workup would include a CBC count and liver function tests (LFTs). Below are listed the prices for some common laboratory tests that might be ordered:**

| | |
|---|---|
| **CBC with differential** | **$ 49** |
| **Sedimentation rate** | **27** |
| **SMA 12/60\*** | **200** |
| **ALT\*** | **19** |
| **GGPT\*** | **28** |

*\*SMA = sequential multiple analyzer; ALT= alanine amino transferase; GGPT = gamma glutamyl transferase. .*

**Imaging tests are not indicated at this time.**

The laboratory studies reveal elevated LFTs. How will you follow-up? Estimate the cost for your workup.

**Assuming that the LFT results are consistent with hepatitis (increased SGPT and SGOT), you would order a hepatitis panel to determine if a virus is causing the hepatitis. This panel consists of:**

| | |
|---|---|
| **HBsAg** | **$44** |
| **HBsAb** | **39** |
| **HBcAb** | **39** |
| **HAA** | **39** |
| **HCA** | **39** |

**If the results are consistent with cholelithiasis (increased alkaline phosphatase and bilirubin), you would obtain a gallbladder ultrasound (cost: $266).**

Gallstones are detected, but the patient does not want surgery as he is worried about having an ugly scar and he has no sick time days at his work. He will have to use his vacation time to have the operation. **You recommend laparoscopic surgery, as it leaves a much smaller scar, costs less (estimate cost: $4800), and he will only miss a few days of work compared to the several weeks usually lost after undergoing a traditional cholecystectomy. Estimate the cost, including the surgeon's fee: $8460. Asymptomatic gallstones do not necessarily need to be removed.**

## Case 6

Anthony, an 8-year-old patient, comes into your office complaining of shortness of breath and wheezing. After your thorough examination, the findings of which are essentially normal other than scattered rhonchi and diffuse wheezing, you decide to order some diagnostic tests. Choose the tests you would order from the list below; estimate the cost.

| Test | Cost |
|------|------|
| _____ Pulmonary function test | $435 |
| _____ Chest x-ray | $169 |
| _____ CBC count | $ 23 |
| _____ Allergy testing | $183 |
| _____ Blood gas | $101 |
| _____ Oxygen saturation | $ 52 |

What is your diagnosis? What will you prescribe? Estimate the cost for your therapy.

**Given the fact that he is otherwise well and that you will be available for follow-up, no testing is necessary at this time. A peak flow performed in the office would be useful to determine how compromised his breathing is. Additionally, he could be given a beta-agonist breathing treatment, with either a nebulizer or inhaler, and re-examined to see if he is improved. You can make a diagnosis of bronchospasm, with the possibility of a viral infection as the etiology, and consider the possibility that he has asthma.**

If you decide to prescribe an inhaler, write the prescription below:

---

**MED STUDENT ASSOCIATES**
**Not for Real Drugs**

NAME:  Anthony                          AGE:      8

ADDRESS:                                DATE:

RX: **Albuterol inhaler #1**
    **Sig: 2 puffs q4–6h prn wheeze**

DEA# _____                              M.D.
                           PHYSICIAN'S SIGNATURE
                           Interchange is mandated unless the practitioner
                           writes the words "no substitution" in this space.

Repeat ___2___ Times
          _____ Month

---

**Appropriate therapy would be to prescribe a beta-agonist inhaler like albuterol. An 8-year-old should be able to use an inhaler but needs to be instructed in its appropriate use. Additional measures would be to recommend follow-up if the patient is not improved or if wheezing persists. The prices for some inhalers are listed in Table A.2.**

The patient returns with continued wheezing. His mother requests allergy-testing as she is concerned that their new cat may be causing the problem, so you refer him for allergy-testing. Estimate the cost for a standard skin-patch test for environmental allergens: **$183**.

The patient tests positive for feline allergy, and you place him on immunotherapy—monthly injections of cat allergen to diminish his allergic response. Estimate the annual cost for his allergy immunotherapy: **$330**.

**At this point one can be comfortable with the diagnosis of asthma. Depending on the severity of his symptoms, pulmonary function tests can be performed. Having the patient learn to use a peak-flow meter at home to monitor his therapy is an inexpensive way to follow progress. (The treatment of asthma is beyond the scope of this workbook.) Environmental control of allergens is a key part of treating chronic asthma. For the patient with confirmed**

## COST OF SOME AEROSOLS FOR ASTHMA

| Drug | Dosage | Canister size (gm) | Contents (puffs) | Cost[a] |
|---|---|---|---|---|
| **Beta-adrenergics** | | | | |
| Albuterol – | | | | |
| (*Proventil* – Schering-Plough) | 2 puffs (90 µg/puff) q4–6h | 17 | 200 | $ 22.06 |
| (*Ventolin* – Allen & Hanburys) | 2 puffs (90 µg/puff) q4–6h | 17 | 200 | 22.06 |
| (*Ventolin Rotacaps*[b]) | 1–2 caps (200 µg/cap) q4–6h | | | 26.02 |
| Bitolterol (*Tornalate* – Dura) | 2–3 puffs (370 µg/puff) q4–6h | 16.4 | 300 | 32.65 |
| Pirbuterol (*Maxair* – 3M) | 2 puffs (200 µg/puff) q4–6h | 25.6 | 300 | 21.96 |
| Salmeterol (*Serevent* – Allen & Hanburys) | 2 puffs (21 µg/puff) q12h | 13 | 120 | 47.95 |
| Terbutaline (*Brethaire* – Geigy) | 2–3 puffs (200 µg/puff) q4–6h | 10.5 | 300 | 19.95 |
| **Corticosteroids** | | | | |
| Beclomethasone dipropionate – | | | | |
| (*Beclovent* – Allen & Hanburys) | 2 puffs (42 µg/puff) qid or 4 puffs bid | 16.8 | 200 | 28.72 |
| (*Vanceril* – Schering-Plough) | 2 puffs (42 µg/puff) qid or 4 puffs bid | 16.8 | 200 | 28.72 |
| Flunisolide (*Aerobid* – Forest) | 2–4 puffs (250 µg/puff) bid | 7 | 100 | 45.32 |
| Triamcinolone acetonide – | 2 puffs (100 µg/puff) | 20 | 240 | 39.84 |
| (*Azmacort* – Rhône-Poulenc Rorer) | tid–qid or 4 puffs bid | | | |
| Cromolyn sodium (*Intal* – Fisons) | 2–4 puffs (800 µg/puff) qid | 14.2 | 200 | 58.10 |
| (*Intal* Nebulizer Solution[c]) | 20 mg qid | | | 48.25 |
| Nedocromil (*Tilade* – Fisons) | 2 puffs (1.75 mg/puff) q6h | 16.2 | 112 | 26.15 |

■ **Table A.2**

[a] *Cost of the canister to the pharmacist, based on Average Wholesale Price listings in* Red Book Update, *April 1994.*
[b] *Each kit contains 96 (200 µg) capsules and a Rotahaler device.*
[c] *Available in 60-ampule packages; each 2-ml ampule contains 20 mg.*
*Source: Drugs for asthma.* Med Lett Drugs Ther 1995; 37:1.

environmental allergies, decreasing exposure to these allergies can save considerable morbidity and expense in physician visits and medication costs.

## Case 7

You are seeing Kate, a 26-year-old previously healthy student who has had symptoms of dysuria and frequency for two days. She denies other problems and her last menstrual period was 1 week ago. On examination, she is afebrile, without flank tenderness, and otherwise appears well. What workup will you obtain? Estimate the cost.

**A microscopic urinalysis in your office can reveal pyuria and may be sufficient to make a diagnosis. Alternatively, you can order a urinalysis (cost: $27) plus a culture and sensitivity test (cost: $91).**

**A recent, elegant article by Barry et al., published in the January 1997 Journal of Family Practice outlines a cost-utility analysis of how to workup and treat such a patient. Empiric treatment without any workup gives the best cost-utility ratio. This excellent article points out the considerations involved in providing cost-effective care.**

What diagnosis are you considering? What therapy will you prescribe? Estimate the cost.

**The presentation is consistent with a diagnosis of cystitis. Single-dose therapy with two tablets of Bactrim DS (trimethoprim-sulfamethoxazole) is appropriate. The cost is $1.42 per day. Table A.3 list the costs of some commonly prescribed antibiotics to treat a urinary tract infection.**

The patient returns monthly with recurrent urinary tract infections. Given this chronic course, what further workup will you order, and what further treatment will you suggest? Again, estimate the cost.

**Initially, securing additional history from the patient is appropriate. The patient should be educated about proper hygiene, postcoital voiding, etc. The patient also should be placed on chronic suppressive therapy with an inexpensive antibiotic like Gantrisin (sulfisoxazole) once a day. If the patient continues to have infections, a more extensive**

## DOSAGE AND COST OF SOME DRUGS FOR TREATMENT OF URINARY TRACT INFECTIONS

| Drug | Dosage | Cost[a] |
|------|--------|---------|
| Amoxicillin – generic price<br>(*Amoxil* – SmithKline Beecham) | 250 mg tid *x* 3 d | $    .70<br>1.94 |
| Cefixime (*Suprax* – Lederle) | 400 mg once *x* 3 d | 21.63 |
| Ciprofloxacin (*Cipro* – Bayer) | 100 mg bid *x* 3 d | 14.40 |
| Enoxacin (*Penetrex* – Rhône-Poulenc Rorer) | 200 mg bid *x* 3 d | 17.12 |
| Fosfomycin (*Monurol* – Forest) | 3 gm once[b] | 25.25 |
| Lomefloxacin (*Maxaquin* – Searle) | 400 mg once *x* 3 d | 19.81 |
| Nitrofurantoin – generic price<br>(*Macrodantin* – Procter & Gamble)<br>(*Macrobid* – Procter & Gamble) | 50 mg qid *x* 7 d<br><br>100 mg bid *x* 7 d | 16.68<br>22.52<br>19.37 |
| Norfloxacin (*Noroxin* – Roberts) | 400 mg bid *x* 3 d | 17.00 |
| Ofloxacin (*Floxin Uropak* – Ortho) | 200 mg bid *x* 3 d | 18.35 |
| Trimethoprim – generic price<br>(*Trimpex* – Roche) | 200 mg once *x* 3 d | .73<br>4.15 |
| Trimethoprim-sulfamethoxazole[c] – generic price<br>(*Bactrim DS* – Roche)<br>(*Septra DS* – Glaxo-Wellcome) | 1 DS tablet bid *x* 3 d | .54<br><br>7.51<br>7.59 |

■ **Table A.3**

[a] *Cost to the pharmacist based on wholesale price (HCFA or AWP) listings in* Drug Topics Red Book *1997 and July* Update. *Other cephalosporins may also be effective.*

[b] *Each single-dose sachet contains 3 grams of fosfomycin. The granules are dissolved in 1/2 cup of water, and taken immediately.*

[c] *Each DS (double-strength) tablet contains 160 mg trimethoprim and 800 mg sulfamethoxazole.*

*Source: Fosfomycin for urinary tract infections.* Med Lett *1997;39:67.*

workup with an intravenous pyelogram (IVP) (cost: $411) and voiding cystogram (cost: $375) should be considered.

## Case 8

Mary, a 39-year-old secretary, presents with complaints of severe headaches. She has been a patient of yours for a long time and you have seen her for routine care and episodic problems. She complained of a similar headache 3 years previously, but it had resolved and this is essentially a new complaint for her. She notes that the headaches are pounding in nature and seem to settle around her eyes, although frequently it seems as though she has a tight band around her head. She points to a spot on the back of her skull where the pain seems particularly severe. The headaches have occurred almost daily over the last couple of weeks. On further questioning, she reports that she does not awaken with the headaches; they seem to come on gradually during the day and are particularly severe by the end of the work day. She goes home and takes some aspirin, which provides minimal relief. Mary is able to get to sleep without difficulty and sleeps through the night. Indeed, she relates that rather than the headaches keeping her up, she feels exhausted at the end of the day and has no problem falling asleep. Her review of systems is otherwise negative. She denies any visual changes, numbness, or weakness. The results of physical examination are essentially within normal limits, with cranial nerves being intact and a funduscopic examination demonstrating normal findings. What diagnostic and/or therapeutic modalities will you employ at this point? Estimate the costs.

**The patient's presentation is consistent with muscle-tension headaches. No diagnostic testing is necessary at this point. She should be prescribed a nonsteroidal anti-inflammatory drug (NSAID) to relieve pain and counseled in simple tension-reducing measures, such as taking frequent short breaks from typing; stretching; and range-of-motion exercises for her neck; massage; and exploration of issues involved in causing stress.**

The patient returns for follow-up in 2 weeks. She reports that the medication you prescribed has helped in relieving the headaches; however, she is concerned that she continues to have them daily. At this point, she expresses her worries about the possibility of a brain tumor and requests that some x-rays be taken or a brain scan performed to be sure that this is not the case. Estimate the cost of a computed tomography (CT) scan of the head: <u>**$605**</u>; or MRI scan of the brain: <u>**$1,437**</u>. What will you do now?

**It is appropriate to repeat the physical examination, including a complete neurologic examination. Additionally, with a description that sounds like muscle-tension headaches, your history should focus on stresses in the patient's life. Quite likely, there is increasing stress at work, given the nature of these headaches and their onset during the day. It is unnecessary to perform a scan when the patient has normal results on physical examination (including vital signs and neurologic findings) and intact cognition, or if the symptoms are not worsening under observation. Studies have shown that the incidence of serious intercranial disease in patients presenting with a new headache is 0.35%. Given such a low incidence in the patient with essentially normal findings, further workup is unnecessary. Should patients have abnormalities on examination or describe the headache as the "worst ever" and if it seems to get worse under observation, then an imaging study would be appropriate.**

**The patient should be reassured. This patient, like many, came in requesting or even demanding a scan. A recent study conducted by the American Academy of Neurology found that the most common benefit from a brain scan was relief of anxiety in the patient. However, this needs to be tempered with disadvantages, such as allergic reactions to the contrast agent, claustrophobic anxiety from the examination, and cost. It does not take an expensive high-tech procedure to reassure patients. Careful listening to their concerns, a thorough physical examination, and then spending time to explain your thinking will alleviate fears and anxiety as well as would doing a scan. It is**

important also to offer patients close follow-up so that they understand that you are taking their complaints seriously and will continue to assess the situation over time.

## Case 9

You are taking care of Peter, a 33-year-old horticultural executive who comes in to see you complaining of what he describes as heartburn. On further questioning, you learn that he has a sharp burning sensation in his epigastrium and substernally. Occasionally, he has a sour taste in the back of his mouth. His symptoms are so severe that they occasionally wake him up from sleep, for which he gets up and has a glass of warm milk and the symptoms seem to resolve. He notes there has been increasing pressure at work, and he has been exploring starting his own business. He otherwise feels well and other than having been seen in the past for routine health visits, his past medical history is benign. He denies problems with vomiting, or diarrhea, or melena. He keeps fit as he has a physically demanding job. He does admit to drinking several cans of Coke on a daily basis and occasionally has a beer or two prior to retiring in the evening. His alcohol intake has increased as of late, as he has begun a new hobby of making his own home brew.

His vital signs are normal. The results of a physical examination are within normal limits, but there is some mild tenderness to palpation over the epigastrium. Given the history and results of physical examination, you feel quite comfortable that his symptoms are not cardiac in nature but limited to the gastrointestinal tract. What diagnostic and therapeutic measures will you undertake at this time? Estimate the cost.

**The patient's presentation is consistent with gastro-esophageal reflux disease, a fairly common ailment. There is no need to undertake any diagnostic testing at this point. The patient should be instructed to avoid caffeinated beverages and alcohol, not to eat after his evening meal, and to avoid milk products. Although milk products have been prescribed in the past because of the calcium's**

141

antacid effect, we now know that calcium can cause or pre-
cipitate a rebound hyperacidic state following its use.
Instead, it would be reasonable to advise the patient to use
over-the-counter antacids such as Maalox or Mylanta for
his complaints.  Additionally, should the symptoms persist
when he is laying down at night, an additional measure
would be for the patient to put 4- to 6-inch wooden blocks
underneath the head of the bed, to raise his head slightly
while he sleeps.

The efficacy of these fairly straightforward and simple
measures should be evaluated in one month to see
whether the patient has been able to adhere to your recommendations and to see if his condition has improved.
Should symptoms continue despite compliance with these
measures, it would be appropriate to prescribe an $H_2$
blocker (Table A.4).  The patient could then be seen in
follow-up in 1 month.  If the patient's condition is not
improved or if the symptoms persist, it would be reasonable to pursue further diagnostic testing to visualize the
upper gastrointestinal tract to confirm diagnosis and rule
out more severe conditions.  Upper gastrointestinal series:
$435; endoscopy $380.

## Drugs for Peptic Ulcers

| Drug | Dosage | Cost[a] |
|---|---|---|
| **H$_2$-receptor antagonists** | | |
| Cimetidine | 400 mg bid | |
| generic price | | $ 23.72 |
| (*Tagamet* – SK Beecham) | | 96.30 |
| Famotidine (*Pepcid* – Merck) | 20 mg bid | 95.85 |
| Nizatidine (*Axid* – Lilly) | 150 mg bid | 96.00 |
| Ranitidine (*Zantac* – Glaxo) | 150 mg bid | 95.66 |
| **Proton-pump inhibitors** | | |
| Lansoprazole (*Prevacid* – TAP) | 15 mg once | 100.75 |
| Omeprazole (*Prilosec* – Astra Merck) | 20 mg once | 108.90 |
| **Other drugs** | | |
| Sucralfate (*Carafate* – Marion Merrell Dow) | 1 gm qid | 91.96 |
| Misoprostol[b] (*Cytotec* – Searle) | 200 µg qid | 88.16 |
| **Antacids** | | |
| Magnesium hydroxide/ aluminum hydroxide/ simethicone | | |
| (*Maalox Extra Strength Antacid* – Ciba) | 15 mL qid | 24.74 |
| (*Mylanta Double Strength* – J & J Merck) | 2 tab qid | 19.12 |

■ **Table A.4**

[a] *Cost to the pharmacist for 30 days' treatment based on wholesale price (AWP) listings in* Drug Topics Red Book Update, *November 1996.*
[b] *FDA-approved only for prevention of NSAID-associated gastric ulcers.*
*Source: Drugs for treatment of peptic ulcers.* Med Lett Drugs Ther *1997; 39:3.*

# B. BOARD REVIEW QUESTIONS

**1.** What percentage of national health-care spending goes to pay for physician services?

   a. 10%

   b. 20%

   c. 40%

   d. 60%

   e. 80%

**2.** Medicare is:

   a. A private health insurance system for the poor and disabled, subsidized by the federal government.

   b. A public health insurance system for the poor and disabled, financed by the state and federal taxes.

   c. A federal health insurance system for the elderly, financed by payroll deductions, with additional payments by those covered.

   d. A federal health insurance system for the poor elderly, financed by payroll deductions.

**3.** What percentage of all health-care spending in the United States is currently financed by the government (local, state, and federal)?

   a. 10%

   b. 20%

   c. 40%

   d. 60%

   e. 80%

4. Medicaid is:

    a. A private health insurance system for the poor and disabled, subsidized by the federal government.

    b. A public health insurance system for the poor and disabled, financed by state and federal taxes.

    c. A federal health insurance system for the elderly, financed by payroll deductions, with additional payments by those covered.

    d. A federal health insurance system for the poor elderly, financed by payroll deductions.

5. Capitated plans reimburse primary care physicians via:

    a. Fee for service, where the physician is paid a prenegotiated fee for every office visit or procedure.

    b. A system based on a negotiated amount of payment per member per month, whether the patient is seen or not.

    c. A system whereby the physician is paid a contracted amount for total care of a panel of patients.

    d. A resource-based relative value system where the physician is paid a set amount depending on the resources used to treat the patient.

6. Diagnostic related groups (DRGs) are:

    a. A system for keeping track of patient records to be used for quality assurance and utilization review practices.

    b. Used for reimbursing physicians based on a set amount, depending on the patient's diagnosis.

    c. A system developed under the Medicare program for reimbursing hospitals for services provided.

    d. A cataloging system used by hospitals that participate in clinical research funded by the National Institutes of Health.

## Answers for Board Review Questions

1. b
2. c
3. c
4. b
5. b
6. c

# C. HOSPITAL COSTS*

| Patient Care | Cost ($) |
|---|---|
| Room and board<br>  Private room<br>  Semiprivate room | <br>575/day<br>550/day |
| Room charge, intensive care unit | 1400/day |
| Total parenteral nutrition (TPN) | 120–600/day |
| TPN nutritional consult | 150 |
| Feeding tube | 38 |
| Physical therapy/15 minutes | 25 |
| Occupational therapy/15 minutes | 22 |
| Respiratory therapy/15 minutes | 60 |
| Ventilator/8 hours | 415 |
| Oxygen therapy, continuous | 113/day |
| Multilumen catheter | 206 |
| Pain service after surgery | 200 |

*This is a partial listing of average costs associated with inhospital patient care.

# D. DIAGNOSTIC IMAGING CHARGES

| Type | Hospital and Physician Charges |
|---|---|
| **Plain Films** | |
| Skull, 1 | $169.00 |
| Sinus film | 220.00 |
| Chest (posteroanterior and lateral) | 169.00 |
| Ribs, 1 side | 274.00 |
| Spine | 162.00 |
| Scoliosis series | 333.00 |
| Hip | 208.00 |
| Abdomen (kidney and urinary bladder) | 223.00 |
| **Contrast Studies** | |
| Upper GI series | 435.00 |
| Barium enema | 501.00 |
| Intravenous pyelogram (IVP) | 411.00 |
| Arthrogram (knee) | 643.00 |
| Carotid arteriogram, 2 sides | 1979.00 |
| Abdominal aortogram | 1260.00 |
| **Miscellaneous** | |
| Magnetic resonance imaging (all types) | 1437.00 |
| Ultrasound (all types) | 266.00 |
| Computed tomography: | |
|   Head without contrast | 605.00 |
|   Head with contrast | 792.00 |
| Chest, without contrast | 728.00 |
| Mammography, 1–2 films | 251.00 |
| Impedance plethysmography (IPG) test | 77.00 |
| Duplex scan | 220.00 |
| Lung scan | 559.90 |
| Kidney scan | 529.10 |

# E. CLINICAL PATHOLOGY DIAGNOSTIC TEST COSTS ($)

| Chemistry | | Hematology | |
|---|---|---|---|
| Amylase | 28 | CBC count | 23 |
| Electrolytes | 46 | Differential | 26 |
| Potassium | 11 | PT | 28 |
| Alkaline phosphatase | 19 | PTT | 36 |
| ALT (SGPT) | 19 | ESR, Westergren | 27 |
| AST (SGOT) | 19 | **Blood Bank** | |
| GGPT | 28 | Red cells processing | 90 |
| Total bilirubin | 19 | Blood X match | 64 |
| LDH | 28 | Blood processing fee | 90 |
| BUN (urea nitrogen) | 13 | Blood administration | |
| HBsAb | 39 | supplies | 90 |
| HBsAg | 44 | Blood-drawing charge | 14 |
| Antinuclear antibody | 39 | Blood type | 22 |
| Rheumatoid fracture | 61 | Antibody screen | 37 |
| Vitamin B12 | 97 | Coombs' direct | 26 |
| Folate | 97 | Fresh-frozen plasma | 101 |
| Arterial blood gas | 101 | Red blood cells | 224 |
| Urinary hCG | 49 | Rh type | 22 |
| Total protein | 19 | **Drug Levels** | |
| Cholesterol | 21 | Digoxin | 92 |
| Creatinine | 13 | Dilantin | 76 |
| Glucose | 13 | Gentamycin | 88 ea |
| SMA-12 | 200 | peak and trough | |
| Transferrin | 75 | **Microbiology** | |
| T3, T4, FT1 | 228 | Blood culture | 85 |
| Serum TSH | 168 | Sputum culture | 49 |
| Urinalysis | 27 | Urine culture | 49 |
| CPK | 28 | Antibiotic sensitivity | 42 |
| RPR test | 29 | Stool ova/parasite | 49 |
| CPK-MB | 41 | examination | |
| PSA | 87 | | |

# F. MISCELLANEOUS CHARGES

| Treatment/Procedure | Approximate Charges ($) |
|---|---|
| Physical therapy/15 minutes | 34 |
| Occupational therapy/15 minutes | 32 |
| Routine audiology evaluation, adult | 75 |
| Behavioral audiometry, child | 50 |
| Tympanostomy with general anesthesia, physician | 380 |
| Flexible sigmoidoscopy to midsigmoid loop with Biopsy | 321 |
| Colonoscopy, average | 625 |
| Endoscopy | 380 |
| Renal dialysis, 2–3/week | 270/month |
| **Cardiology** | |
| EKG | 86 |
| Cardiac nutritional evaluation | 81 |
| Echocardiogram | 500 |
| Stress test, treadmill/bicycle | 532 |
| Myocardial imaging (thallium), stress/rest | 1660 |
| Percutaneous transluminal coronary angioplasty | 5676 |
| Cardiac catheterization, right and left | 3752 |
| **Ambulance Service** | |
| Nonemergent discharge trip from hospital to anywhere with basic life support, private | 225 + 5–10¢/mile |
| Emergent service with advanced life support and paramedics, private | 300–400 + 5–10¢/mile |
| Helicopter transportation fee | 1999 |
| Professional transportation fee (for helicopter) | 1560 |

| Treatment/Procedure | Approximate Charges ($) |
|---|---|
| **Pulmonary Function Tests** | |
| Routine | 435 |
| **Allergy Tests** | |
| Skin-patch test, 4 panels | 183 |
| Allergy immunotherapy, e.g., cat allergen | 150/year |

# G. PHYSICIAN FEE FOR SELECTED PROCEDURES

| Procedure | National Median | National Range |
|---|---|---|
| **Nonsurgical** | | |
| Flexible sigmoidoscopy | $ 150 | $   50–275 |
| Newborn examination | 130 | 60–200 |
| Spinal tap | 141 | 80–300 |
| EMG | 165 | 90–300 |
| Individual psychotherapy (45 min) | 115 | 80–175 |
| Endoscopy | 475 | 300–650 |
| **Surgical** | | |
| Newborn circumcision | 135 | 60–200 |
| Hysterectomy | 2100 | 1000–4000 |
| Normal OB care, complete | 2100 | 1200–3500 |
| OB care with C-section | 2500 | 1400–4000 |
| D&C | 570 | 300–900 |
| Appendectomy | 1050 | 600–1600 |
| Laparoscopic cholecystectomy | 2100 | 1000–3000 |
| Routine cholecystectomy | 1880 | 1000–2200 |
| Hernia repair | 1000 | 600–1400 |
| Hip replacement | 4200 | 2500–6000 |
| CABG x 3 | 5400 | 3000–9000 |

# INDEX